The Sirtfood Diet Recipes Book

The Only 40 Effective Recipes to Activate Sirtuins

The Cookbook to Lose Weight, Burn Fat and Stay Fit.

BY

Adele Green

Table of Contents

INTRODUCTION 1

What is the Sirtfood diet? 2

On The Sirtfood Diet What Can You Eat? 5

Is It Effective? 6

Is It Sustainable And Healthy? 9

Safety, And Side Effects. 11

How to Adopt the Sirtfood Diet. 13

Top Foods for Men. 17

Healthy Nutrition For Women. 31

Weight Loss and Your Health. 41

Myths About Weight Loss 54

Keys To Change Your Diet To A Successful Weight Loss Over The Long Term 74

Easy and Delicious SirtFood Recipes. 86

Sirtfood Green Juice 86

Shredded Chicken Bowl 89

Buckwheat and Nut Loaf 92

Sweet Potato and Salmon Patties 94

Butterbean and Vegetable Korma 98

Baked salmon with stir fried vegetables 100

Lemon paprika chicken with vegetables........102

Sirtfood Bites 104

Raw carrot and almond loaf 106

Savoury Seed Truffles................................107

Courgette Tortilla 109

Asian king prawn stir-fry with buckwheat
noodles..110

Polenta Bake 112

Buckwheat Pancakes 114

Pea, Miso and Mint Soup 115

Buckwheat Kasha with Mushrooms and Onions
....116

Sirt Muesli 119

Buckwheat Noodle and Green Bean Soup......120

Sirtfood Diet's smoked salmon omelette 121

Chicken breast with kale,red onions, a tomato
and chilli salsa 122

Cauliflower and Chickpea Masala 124

Sirtfood bites..127

Sirt Super Salad..129

Sirtfood Diet's Shakshuka........................130

Green Bean,Tomato and Almond Stir Fry......132

Iced Coconut Matcha Latte......................134

Pear Salad with Avocado, Walnuts,and Grilled Chicken 136

Maple Balsamic Dressing 137

Moong Dahl 139

Dill roasted mackerel with tomatoes & steamed vegetables 141

Quinoa, Edamame and Pomegranate Seed Pilaf 142

Quinoa Risotto with Tofu and Asparagus. 144

Buckwheat Bean and Tomato Risotto 145

Asian Shrimp Stir-Fry With Buckwheat Noodles 146

Sirtfood Diet's turmeric baked salmon 148

Strawberry Buckwheat Tabbouleh 150

Vegan Carrot Ginger Soup (Instant Pot) 151

Aromatic Chicken Breast With Kale & Red Onions And A Tomato And Chili Salsa 153

Miso-Marinated Baked Cod With Stir-Fried Greens & Sesame 155

CONCLUSION **157**

INTRODUCTION

Sirtfoods are a recently discovered group of nutrient-rich foods that appear to be able to ' activate ' the body's skinny genes (also known as sirtuins), in much the same way as fasting diets do, with the same set of benefits but without the typical downsides of fasting diets such as irritability, hunger and muscle loss.

By eating a diet rich in Sirtfoods, participants are claimed to lose weight, gain muscle, look and feel better and perhaps even live a longer and healthier life.

It is a diet that is hailed as the next 5:2 and has a whole host of celebrities promoting this. The Sirtfood Diet is not just about weight loss (although that can happen!), but also about improving overall health and well-being, longevity and resistance to disease.

What is the Sirtfood diet?

It's everyone's talking about the latest diet craze, a diet rich in' sirt foods.' These special foods work, according to researchers, by activating specific proteins in the body, called sirtuins. Sirtuins are thought to protect the body's cells from dying when under stress, and are thought to regulate inflammation, metabolism, and aging. Scientists also conclude that sirtuins affect the capacity of the body to burn fat and improve the metabolism, resulting in a weight loss of seven pounds a week while retaining muscle.

Nutritionists Aiden Goggins and Glen Matten created The Sirtfood Diet. They were so interested in Sirtfoods ' ability, they developed a diet based on optimizing the intake of Sirtfood and limiting mild calories. They then tested this diet on an exclusive London gym participants and were surprised by their findings. In the first 7 days gym members lost an average of 7lbs, despite not rising their exercise levels. The participants not only lost a substantial amount of weight, but also gained muscle (usually the opposite happens while dieting) and showed significant improvements in overall health and well-being.

The diet.

So what are the magic' sirtfoods'? The ten most frequently used include: green tea, dark chocolate (that is at least 85% cocoa), apples, blueberries, capers, citrus fruits, parsley, red wine, turmeric, kale the diet is a two-phase approach; the initial phase in lasts one week and involves a three-day reduction of calories to 1000kcal consuming three sirtfood green juices & one meal per day.

The juices include kale, green tea and lemon, celery, rocket, parsley, and meals include buckwheat fry turkey escalope with basil, chicken and kale curry, capers and parsley, and prawn stir fry.

Intakes are increased from days four to seven to 1500kcal consisting of two sirtfood green juices and two sirtfood-rich meals a day.

The second phase is known as the 14 day maintenance phase where there is a steady weight loss. The writers think it's a practical and safe way to lose weight. Focusing on weight loss, though, is not what the diet is about–it's supposed to be about consuming the best food that nature has to offer. I suggest three healthy sirtfood-rich meals a day along with one sirtfood-green juice over the long term.

On The Sirtfood Diet What Can You Eat?

The diet system, as illustrated in The Official Sirtfood Diet, is based on a meal plan that is designed to be full of sirt foods, but curtailed in total calorie counts. Yes, according to the New York Post, one of the writers of the book says it may help you lose seven pounds in a single week. But the meal plan for the book is quite regimented: Dieters are supposed to eat just 1,000 calories per day for the first three days, consisting of a single meal and two green juices. Dieters will enjoy 1,500-cal meal plans for four days later in the first week which are mostly split between two meals.

Most of the plan asks dietarians to build high in sirt foods meals... And not so much. Some of the staples illustrated by the diet include many different items to eat, including kale, tomatoes, onions, parsley, arugula, blueberries and capers. Many grains are highly praised, such as buckwheat, and walnuts, as are spices like turmeric. It is interesting to note that beverages such as coffee, matcha green tea and red wine are encouraged, as is a heavy reliance on 85% dark chocolate.

Is It Effective?

The Sirtfood Diet's authors make bold claims, including that the diet can cause super-charge weight loss, turn your "skinny gene" on and prevent disease.

There is no convincing evidence that the Sirtfood Diet has a more beneficial effect on weight loss than any other diet limited by calories.

And although many of those foods have medicinal properties, no long-term human studies have been conducted to assess if eating a diet rich in sirt foods has any measurable health benefits.

Nonetheless, a pilot study carried out by the authors and involving 39 participants from their fitness center is recorded in the Sirtfood Diet book. The results of this study/research do not seem to have been published elsewhere.

Participants followed the diet for a week and were exercising daily. Participants lost an average of 7pounds (3.2 kg) at the end of the week, and retained or even added muscle mass. However, these findings are hardly shocking. Limiting your calorie intake to 1,000 calories, and actively exercising, will almost always cause weight loss.

Nonetheless, this kind of rapid weight loss is neither real nor long-lasting, and after the first week, this study did not follow participants to see if they gained any of the weight back, which is usually so.

As well as burning fat and muscle, when your body is deprived of energy, it uses its emergency energy stores, or glycogen.

Each glycogen molecule requires 3–4 water molecules for storage. When your body uses glycogen, that water also gets rid of it. It is known as the "water weight." Only about 1/3 of the weight loss comes from fat during the first week of intense calorie restriction, while the other two-thirds come from skin, muscle and glycogen.

The body must replenish its glycogen stores as soon as the calorie intake rises, and the weight comes right back.

However, this form of calorie restriction can also cause your body to reduce its metabolic rate, causing energy requirements to be even lower in calories per day.

This diet is likely to help you lose a few pounds in the beginning, but it'll probably return as soon as the diet is over.

As for the prevention of diseases, it is likely three weeks not long enough to have any meaningful long-term effects.

In this case, it may very well be a good idea to add sirtfood to your regular diet over the long term. But you might as well skip the diet in that case, and start doing it now.

Is It Sustainable And Healthy?

Sirtfoods are almost all healthy choices, and due to their antioxidant or anti-inflammatory properties, they can even produce some health benefits.

Yet eating only a handful of particularly healthy foods can not satisfy all the nutritional needs of your body.

The Sirtfood Diet is unnecessarily restrictive and does not offer any clear, unique health advantages over any other diet.

Additionally, eating only 1,000 calories is not typically recommended without a doctor's supervision. For many people, only eating 1,500 calories per day is overly restrictive.

In addition, the diet requires up to three green juices per day. Though juices may be a good source of vitamins and minerals, they are also a sugar source and almost contain none of the nutritious fibers that whole fruits and vegetables do.

What's more, all-day sipping on juice is a bad idea for both your blood sugar and your teeth.

Not to mention, since the diet is so limited in calories and food choices, protein, vitamins and minerals are more than likely deficient, especially during the first phase.

This diet can be difficult to stick to for the entire three weeks due to the low calorie levels and restrictive food choices.

Add that to the high initial cost of buying a juicer, the book and some rare & expensive ingredients, as well as the time cost of preparing different meals and juices, and this diet is unfeasible and unsustainable for some.

The Sirtfood Diet promotes healthy food but is restrictive in choices of calories and foods. It's also involves drinking lots of juice which is not a recommendation for healthy use.

Safety, And Side Effects.

While the first phase of the Sirtfood Diet is very low in calories and nutritionally incomplete, the average, healthy adult has no real safety concerns taking into account the short duration of the diet.

Yet limiting calories and mostly drinking juice for the first few days of the diet can cause dangerous changes in blood sugar levels for someone with diabetes.

However, even a healthy person may experience some side effects— primarily hunger.

Eating only 1,000 calories –1,500 calories per day will leave just about anyone feeling hungry, particularly if much of what you're eating is juice that's low in fiber, a nutrient that helps you stay full.

During phase one, due to the calorie restriction, you might experience other side effects such as fatigue, lightheadedness and irritability.

Serious health effects are impossible for the otherwise healthy adult if the diet is followed for a mere three weeks.

How to Adopt the Sirtfood Diet.

The Sirtfood Diet has two (2) phases that last three weeks altogether. You can then proceed to "sirtify" your diet by including as many sirt foods as possible into your meals.

The meals are full of sirtfoods but in addition to the "top 20 sirtfoods," other ingredients do.

Many sirtfoods and ingredients are easy to find.

Three of the signature ingredients needed for these two phases— matcha green tea powder, lovage, and buckwheat — can, however, be costly or hard to find.

A large part of the diet is its green juice, which you'll have to make between one and three times a day. A juicer (a blender won't work) and a kitchen scale will be required, as the ingredients are described by weight. The recipe underneath is:.

Green Juice syrup.

- 75 Grams Kale (2.5 oz).
- Arugula (rocket) 30 grams (1 oz)
- 5 grams parsley.
- 2 celery sticks.
- Ginger 1 cm (0.5).
- Half of Apple Green.
- half a lemon.
- Half a teaspoon of green Tea matcha.

Juice all ingredients together, except the green tea powder and lemon, and pour them into a glass. Juice the lemon by hand, then stir in both the lemon juice and the green tea powder.

Phase One.

The first process lasts for seven days, with calorie restriction and lots of green juice involved. It's meant to boost your weight loss and claim to help you lose 7 pounds (3.2 kg) in seven days.

Intake of calories during the first three days of phase one is limited to 1,000 calories. You drink three green juices, plus one meal, per day. You can pick from recipes in the book every day, all of which involve sirtfood as a major part of the meal.

Examples of meals include miso-glazed tofu, the omelet sirtfood or a shrimp stir-fry with buckwheat noodles.

Calorie intake is increased to 1,500 on days 4–7 of phase one. It involves two green juices a day and two more sirtfood-rich meals that can be picked from the book.

Phase Two.

Phase two takes two weeks to complete. You should continue to loose weight steadily during this "maintenance" phase.

This step has no clear calorie limit. Alternatively, you eat three sirt-fed meals and one green juice a day.

The meals are again chosen from the supplied recipes.

What happens once you've completed the Sirtfood Diet?

The Sirtfood Diet is not intended as a one-off' diet' but rather as a way of life. You are encouraged to continue eating a diet rich in Sirtfoods once you've completed the first 3 weeks, and continue to drink your daily green juice. The writers of The Sirtfood Diet have continued to release The Sirtfood Diet Recipe Book since they released their original book, with recipes for loads of more syrtfood-rich main meals, as well as recipes for alternatives to green juice and more hints and tips to adopt the Sirtfood Diet. There are even some Sirtfood dessert recipes here! The Sirtfood Diet authors suggest that phases 1 and 2 can be repeated as and when required for a health boost, or if things have gone a little off track.

Top Foods for Men.

The health problems are somewhat different between men and women. We've been hearing so much about women's diet and nutrition and I think it's time for men to check in!
So...... then... Here are some Top Men Foods.

Pumpkin seeds, almonds, Brazils, and Walnuts.

Nuts are often viewed as high-fat foods and are shunned, with little knowledge of their nutritional value. Most nuts are very fatty; Brazil nuts are around 70% fat so you would not want to eat too many at a time, but only 10% of this fat is specifically saturated, so you can see that the vast majority is "unsaturated" and therefore either essential or potentially useful to the health of each cell in the body. In this context, the term "essential" simply means that our bodies don't produce certain fats (especially Omega-3 & Omega-6 fats), which means that the only way to obtain them is through the foods we eat... Necessary to life, and thus necessary to diet! Most fresh unsalted and unroasted nuts and seeds, as well as oily fish such as avocados, vegetable, salmon, and seed oils, and olive oil mostly contain essential fatty acids-in other words, fats that we need and that are put to good use in the body. A handful of walnuts have as many omega-3 fatty acids as 3 ounces of salmon, which may help in light of recent and ongoing concerns over farmed salmon. Not only do omega-3 fats help to prevent heart disease, they also contribute to reducing inflammation and depression.

A 25 g serving of brazils (about 10 nuts) would be an ideal morning snack or addition to cereal or fruit. It would give you 170 kcals, and 17 grams of fat, respectively. Around 70 g of fat in one day is appropriate so they aren't fattening as part of your whole diet! Brazils are one of the mineral selenium's highest food sources: an antioxidant that plays a vital role in the protection of the heart and CV system, as well as the thyroid gland. Selenium is also known to be a potent anticancer agent. Because of a decline in soil levels over the years, and therefore a reduction in crops, British diets still ignore it. All is not lost though if you regularly eat a few Brazils... The 25 g portion above would give you 383 micrograms (ug), way over the 45-75ug UK RNI, so even half that amount would still be beneficial!

Seeds (particularly pumpkin seeds) are significantly lower in fat than nuts; pumpkin seeds are only 45% fat, and again most are unsaturated. They are as well have a higher protein content than many nuts, and also contain more zinc. Nuts still provide a decent source of protein, with the highest amount of almonds and the highest amount of calcium. When it comes to magnesium, another important mineral for men that works closely with calcium in bone and muscle function, Brazil nuts once again top of the list. As you can see, it's variety that counts and it certainly provides the "spice" of life as we know it, but it also provides the key to obtaining the full spectrum of nutrients that we need to be healthy every day.

Did you know?

A sperm body contains monounsaturated fat of 86 per cent! So, healthy sperm require healthy fats (and a good dose of selenium!). Olive oil and macadamia nuts are the foods with the most similar fatty acid profiles to that of sperm, but all the foods above come pretty close too!

Your Prostate and Flaxseeds.

Some recent research has shown people with early stage prostate cancer who eat a low-fat diet plus three tbsps of ground flaxseed per day for just over a month have seen their PSA levels decline. They have also seen their levels of testosterone and cholesterol go down. PSA, or prostate-specific antigen, indicates the growth of the tumour. The men who had more advanced cancers have seen the PSA scores keep rising. But researchers believe that they may have seen some benefit as well had they remained on a flaxseed diet longer.

Flaxseed is high in fiber, lignans and fatty acids of omega-3, all of which can help to fight cancer.

Soya foods.

Versatile soya foods include tofu, soya beans, fermented products like tamari or soy sauce, and miso. They are not only one of the best vegetable protein sources, but soya foods also boast the presence of plant substances called "isoflavones." These have various health benefits for men. Soja protein helps lower the amount of harmful LDL cholesterol in the blood, and soya isoflavones are now considered to protect against prostate cancer, as well as heart disease.

Firm tofu is the most effective way to enjoy the health benefits of soya. Contrary to popular belief, tofu can be really nutritious, and even tasty. Try marinating it in lemon juice, soy sauce, oil, and herbs to get the most out of your tofu and then bake, grill or stir-fry it with your veggy choice.

Quinoa.

Quinoa is a good energy food and definitely in the "Good Men's Foods" list, partially because it has the greatest amino acid profile of all the grains! Which means you can count it in as a decent source of protein, and even better when mixing it with eggs, chicken or fish. It's also packed with vitamins and minerals (especially vitamins B, calcium, and magnesium). Like bananas and avocados, it's also high in potassium, all of which help keep blood pressure within a healthy range. It's very low in fat and completely free of cholesterol, so watching their dietary cholesterol intake is a winner for those concerned.

Eggs.

Eggs (preferably organic wherever possible) are a first-class protein source, easy to cook and an ideal way to start a busy day. A high protein breakfast like scrambled eggs on wholegrain toast efficiently balances blood sugar levels, and will definitely feed you much longer than toast and jam. If you're concerned about the content of eggs with cholesterol, limit your intake to 3 per week; otherwise there's no need to worry. Also the eggs are high in choline (vital to keep the memory boys!!) and the lutein and zeaxanthin carotenoids... These are important for helping to prevent cataracts and age-related macular degeneration, both leading to blindness.

Eggs are easy to cook, really... Hard-boil, soft-boil, poach, scramble them-just try not to cook them with excessive quantities of butter, cream or oil. Benedict eggs should be a treat "once in a while!"

Oysters and other Seafood.

Oysters are rich in the mineral zinc-commonly known as mineral fertility! Oysters are famed for their aphrodisiac reputation, and I guess it is the high content of zinc which gives this reputation many scientific basis? The truth is that oysters do contain an extraordinarily high quantity of zinc-essential for sperm production and reproductive organ development.

Unfortunately, oysters aren't to everyone's taste, so are there any other foods that might have similar effects? Well, some are mentioned above (pumpkin seeds and sunflower seeds) but other excellent dietary zinc sources include, to name a few, crab, most other shellfish, offal and wheatgerm. But I do not think any of those have a reputation for being true aphrodisiacs... Offal and Oyster?

I consider Oysters as for me.... Most preferably with a glass of champagne!

Garlic.

Garlic must be one of the planet's healthiest and most helpful foods / herbs. It is probably one of the oldest cultivated plants, native to Central Asia. It is often spoken of as "anti-aging" since it is an excellent source of antioxidants. Antioxidants literally stop' rusting' or ageing cells. We see this process visibly as rubbish! Garlic is also full of nutrients such as vitamins B, calcium, sulphur and zinc, though in moderate quantities. But what garlic is most renowned for is the anti-bacterial benefits due to the active substance in garlic, called allicin. For this cause garlic is so good of colds and flu. Garlic supplements (which remains stable until dried) will contain the active substance, as it is the allicin properties that help to maintain a healthy heart and circulation, as well as having wonderful anti-microbial activity. Garlic acts in the blood as an anti-coagulant which reduces the risk of strokes and can help destroy cancer cells. RAW, chopped, chopped or pulverized, and added to a salad dressing is the best way to eat garlic? But I must admit "garlic smoke" isn't very attractive!! Tend to chew raw parsley after a heavily laced meal with the garlic. This acts to neutralize the pungent garlic smell, since the parsley chlorophyll acts as a cleanser and neutralizer. The alternative is to take one capsule of garlic daily.

Avocados.

I guess avocados feel a little bit like butter on the tongue, but have a nutty flavour? Spanish sailors actually called them "midshipman's butter," because they used them on long sea trips as a replacement for butter. Avocados contain good quantities of B vitamins, including folate, and are among the few vitamin E-containing fruits. An essential antioxidant soluble in fat. Vitamin E is required to turn cholesterol into male sex hormones and deficiency of vitamin E can cause fertility in both sexes by damaging the reproductive tissue. If you guys all out there... A regular dietary portion of avocado with a handful of sunflower seeds and pumpkin seeds (also high in "E") wouldn't miss your best health!

Surprising to some perhaps, but avocados contain twice as much potassium as bananas, and are a great source of phytochemical lutein... Also found in green leafy vegetables, and a key nutrient to improve eye health. Avocados, like olive oil, provide good, monounsaturated fat, which is crucial in reducing

LDL cholesterol. Giving it a gentle squeeze while checking an "avo" for ripeness-a ripe fruit leaves a finger or thumbprint. To eat avocados, cut lengthwise carefully, and prize away from the stone. Scoop the flesh out, and enjoy! Seek to scramble the green fruit for a beautiful guacamole with chopped tomatoes, lime or lemon juice, a touch of chopped fresh chilli and salt. Mixing with ricotta cheese often Servings: a healthy dip which is super low-fat.

My childhood experience of eating avocados is mixed with fresh whole meal bread and a little salt-delicious!

Bananas and apples.

Apples are packed with several potent antioxidants including a compound called quercetin. Quercetin is considered to be a very effective natural antihistamine which acts synergistically with another antihistamine-vitamin C. During the "allergy" season, fever sufferers in Hay find this combination very useful. You may find supplements that often combine these with bromelain, which is a good anti-inflammatory. Apples also have a high content of soluble fibre, pectin, which helps lower LDL cholesterol. So must the saying "An apple a day keeps the doctor away" have some truth? The best way to eat them is to be ripe, raw and with the peel intact-don't peel apples, as you will find the quercetin in the skin!

Bananas contain tons of potassium, magnesium, and folate (like avocados). Potassium helps to combat high blood pressure and lowers the risk of strokes. A high diet of fruits and vegs should give you plenty of potassium. Folate is essential for proper cell growth, and in the homocysteine in the blood-vital for heart disease prevention.

Berry fruits.

Besides being rich in vitamin C, purple, dark red and blue berries are anti-aging, they can also be beneficial for gout sufferers. Gout is a very distressing condition, and is the result of pouring uric acid into tissues-often in the big toe! This induces inflammation and pain, and may lead to arthritis and joint degeneration. Unfortunately, it's also often related to kidney problems and the risk of kidney stones is increased. Because of the existence of antioxidants such as anthocyanins and proanthocyanins, fruits such as blackberries and blueberries etc. will benefit-this is what gives them such a rich glorious colour. Better yet, they are natural anti-inflammatory drugs so inflammatory pain can be eased. Good sufferers must also follow a low diet of animal protein, limit alcohol, drink plenty of water and eat lots of more colorful fruit and veg.

Oats.

Oats are rich in both B vitamins and calcium, and insoluble and soluble fiber. It means that they are not only safe, they can also help keep the intestines free of toxins-as well as help eliminate waste too!

The high/large content of soluble fibers in oats is the reason why they have been shown to lower levels of

LDL cholesterol (the nasty cholesterol) when consumed regularly. By adding one bowl of porridge oats to your daily diet, you'll do something very important to protect yourself against heart disease. Another great source of linseed soluble fibre, so add a tablespoon to your morning bowl of oats. The best to go for is absolute organic oats!

Healthy Nutrition For Women.

Today is a great time for women as more knowledge based on scientific evidence is emerging from medical science to dispel myths and present facts.

Women's Diets Confusion abounds from anti-heart disease diet to PMS diet to hundreds of diets on weight-loss.

Solution: Women want to simplify the puzzle of nutrition and get one diet. The One Diet is the Diet Plan for the Healthy Woman.

Healthy Woman's diet plan takes into account how the dietary guidelines help prevent one illness, such as heart disease, and how it might communicate with therapy for another condition, such as obesity, food cravings, osteoporosis, diabetes.

Previous trends-Not "Everything in your head"

Women's complaints about wellbeing were ignored as "all in the brain."

"Insecurity, fatigue, irritability the week before menstruation, indicated emotionalism, a desire for sweets, lack of willpower. When these symptoms were mentioned to a physician, a partner or a relative. Their concern met with a smile or suggestion" to take it easy. "Vague signs of lethargy, exhaustion, mood swings, vomiting, and fluid retention were all poor conditions.

Changing Times.

It is now understood that undiagnosed emotional and physical symptoms are particular biochemical processes, many of which are impaired by diet. Mood swings; food cravings and anxiety are signs encountered by many women before their periods and are now called Premenstrual Syndrome (PMS). The diet and exercise changes can partially alleviate

PMS. Low concentration, memory problems and tiredness may result from something as simple as iron deficiency and the intake of caffeine.

Very recently, the unavoidable state of finding love was known to be many diseases: the frail, stooped old lady with a protruding belly was the fate of a woman. Scientists agree this disorder-osteoporosis-can be avoided or at least significantly slowed down by exercise and increasing calcium intake in the diet.

Numerous age-related illnesses may be avoided from cataracts and skin ageing to bowel disorders, heart disease, and many of the menopause-related emotional and physical changes, or symptoms may be decreased by a few dietary changes. With regular exercise in your sixties, seventies and beyond, there's every reason to feel vibrant, radiant and youthful.

What You Can Do To Re-Program The Aging Process!

Getting older is a natural process but you need not succumb to it. Many conditions linked to aging and ill health result from action defenses that could be reinforced by a low-fat, nutrient-dense diet combined with exercise. For example, consuming ample amounts of antioxidant nutrients, including beta-carotene, vitamin C, vitamin E, and selenium, reinforces one of the body's basic anti-aging defense systems.

Optimal consumption of trace minerals, iron, zinc and copper and many of the vitamins strengthen the body's immune system and protect against colds, allergies, premature aging and many diseases like cancer and arthritis.

Fitness.

Staying fit by eating a low-fat, rich diet of nutrients and exercising every day; you can re-program the ageing process of your body. Basically what you eat and how much you move can make the difference between feeling and looking great, or at best just get by while the aging process is progressing towards disease and disability.

Ability to Improve

Your diet has to work for you to improve your health ability, rather than against you. It's not too late to get your diet better. Today the standard for a safe "balanced diet" for women is shifting and some degenerative diseases or emotional problems may not be good to avoid.

Evidence has shown female diets have a long way to go. Women eat less whole milk and beef than women did years ago which lessened saturated fat and cholesterol. The decline in heart disease is 29 per cent. On the other side, polyunsaturated fats such as vegetable oils and margarine have skyrocketed and the recommended amount is less than one-third of the average intake of fiber (i.e. 10 grams versus 30 + grams).

Women eat more chicken than beef but they fry the chicken. (One serving of chicken nuggets is equal to five pats of butter.) Salad consumption is increasing as a result of the search for weight loss, and that is healthy. Nevertheless, high fat salad dressings are poured on them which dilute the benefits. The guidelines for raising complex carbohydrates such as brown rice, pasta, bread and cereals are not followed. Women are still consuming less than half the amount of these foods their forefathers ate in the 1900's. Women eat more French fries cake, sugar, and doughnuts than pasta. Such food choices increase fat and sugar consumption, which challenge the diet's nutritional adequacy.

Jeopardy-The Specifications do not follow.

Women's diets are low in many essential nutrients because they don't eat enough of the recommended diet. Servings of a woman's physiology: her more vulnerable to nutrient deficiencies during various stages of her life, such as puberty, pregnancy and menopause, than a man.

One in two woman consumes less than two-thirds of the Recommended Dietary Allowance (RDI) for folic acid, copper, zinc, calcium, vitamin E, iron, magnesium, vitamin and many of the B vitamins. Many of these shortcomings are caused by eating too many of these processed foods, fast foods, and convenience items which are high in fat and sugar and low in nutrients. It showed that the average women consume 13 teaspoons of sugar per day, or 265 calories from the foods that provide small or no nutritional value.

Women love dieting. In the United States the average diet range for women starts at 1,400 to 1,800 calories. Compare this with men, who usually consume more than 2,500 calories per day, when food intake is restricted to these amounts, it is very impossible to meet the requirement values for all vitamins and minerals.

Clinical problems are not addressed if women don't drink the recommended minimum volume. It further compounds the problem as they don't get the amounts needed to prevent cancer, heart disease, premature aging and other disorders including PMS and osteoporosis. Other nutrients such as beta-carotene and vitamin C are required in quantities greater than previously recognized. If a woman consumes at least 5 servings of fruits and vegetables each day, it can be obtained from the diet. In short, women don't eat enough of the proper food.

What You Can Do.

Women wear many hats and lead very active lives, with jobs, family responsibilities and social responsibility. Given busy lives, women need to take time to look after themselves. There is no such thing as good health. The body is complex and will naturally deteriorate at increasing speed, unless you play a constructive role in managing it well.

Form good habits to support a healthy body, and requires only minor adjustments in a healthy lifestyle in most cases. Such practices are not instinctive. You'll need to pick nutritious foods. You got to make a conscious effort to handle it well by eating nutritious food and setting in motion to support your goals of health and fitness.

One of the most important dietary changes that you can make for your wellbeing, waistline, and beauty is eating less fat and less fibre-rich foods. More fat means more nutrients for every spoonful of food consumed. Less fat signifies a longer, healthier life. It is noticeable that as the population ages, women become more serious about eating for health and sorting to find diets with which they can live through the conflicting noises. Know this, diets don't work at best, and at worst they can endanger health, disease, resistance, and life spans.

It is up to you to become your own advocate of nutrition and note that for many of these disorders the symptoms you experience are not entirely in your head, and that there are physical and probably nutritional bases. However, in an effort to attain and maintain your healthiest body, you are still responsible for taking care of your health and nutritional status.

Weight Loss and Your Health.

Experiencing difficulty in searching for a complete and accurate guide to weight reduction, search no more. This book will take you to a safer and sexier body with the best and most positive acts. Unlike other advices that focus only on a single part of diet, this book will feature all you need to know about weight reduction.

You must first understand how the body process works before entering into any diet or exercise programme. The body has the ability to use a calorie maintenance level to perform its daily function. The proper amount of calories allows you to walk around and maintain internal body functions. Calories are the source of energy for the body. You'll feel sick without the proper amount of calories.

The calories that we need come from our eating and drinking habits. Weight does not go up or down because we eat the same number of calories that match for our daily needs. Demonstrating this explanation: if your maintenance number is 3000 calories, and you eat the same amount a day, your weight will not be increased. Weight increases when we consume more than the level of calories we maintain. The opposite occurs when we use up the daily maintenance level, which is weight loss. We can also reduce calories from our daily maintenance level by eating less. Therefore, an adult with a maintenance quantity of 3000 calories will consume 2500 calories to reduce weight.

I am sure you would want to understand your level of calorie maintenance at this moment. Your maintenance level is calculated using the Harris-Benedict Equation Basel Metabolic Rate (BMR). The BMR of the body is the amount of calories that you need to consume to keep your daily responsibilities performed. How much exercise you do is weighed when measuring the calories that you need to burn per day. Also, you can search for online calculators for daily calorie maintenance level to understand what your body needs.

Now that you've learned the idea behind weight reduction, it's time to know the basic ways of weight loss. Those three essential ways are all you need. The first is to get to work out. Exercise can give you more calories to burn. Unless you stick to the maintenance level of your daily calories you will end up losing the same amount. So no change in weight occurs. But if you'd like to reduce weight, you'll have to engage in exercise that loses a larger amount from your maintenance level of calories. You'll have to cut additional 500 calories for weight loss with the past example.

You will also have to eat less of your daily maintenance number, apart from exercise. Those with a maintenance volume of 3000 will have to lose 500 calories and consume only 2500. There's a caloric deficit as you give your body a smaller amount of the calories it needs for maintenance. Engaging in more caloric shortages will cause a consistent weight loss for the body.

The best and most popular weight-loss method requires both diet and exercise. Eating less calories and burning more calories gives the body a stability of what your activities are gaining and losing. It has been repeatedly established that you will get faster and longer lasting weight loss results through a healthy diet and workouts. Using both approaches is also the best way, and does not mess with your daily responsibilities.

Before jumping into a workout routine or diet, you must first evaluate the maintenance level of your body. The analysis will be the adjustment of your form toward a better routine. Start by regularly eating your calorie maintenance level for each day. Sustain such caloric intake for 2 to 3 weeks. It need not be the same amount of calories as long as it is really close. Weigh yourself once a week (before eating and on an empty stomach) at the start of the day to ensure you are eating the right amount.

If you've had a steady weight for the two to three weeks then you've been able to eat the calories your maintenance standard requires. To may your weight, you will eat 500 less of your daily maintenance amount per day. If your maintenance standard is 2500, you need to start consuming only 2000 calories per day.

Those who were unable to maintain their calories can still start a healthy weight reduction programme. All you have to do is eat 500 less of your maintenance level and redo the body change with the reduced amount of calories. If you have been good in eating the lowered level of maintenance, you will start consuming minus 500 of the initial amount again.

To ensure you don't lose the weight too fast is crucial to one. Reducing weight at a dangerous pace can threaten your well-being. When you find yourself consistently losing three or more pounds for some weeks in a row each week, then you will have to make some adjustments. The adjustment includes 250 to 300 calories to your daily intake. After that, with the new quantity, you have to start observing your weight. You shouldn't eat a smaller amount just remember. For needed enough calories you need to exercise for a healthy weight reduction.

The speed of weight reduction prescribed is around one to two pounds per week. Remember, your body will not benefit from weight reductions very quickly. You have to maintain a loss velocity that will keep you fit. Much more important to your wellbeing than to look good. With very rapid weight loss our bodies can't catch up. In fact, if you quicken the procedure it will simply change to stay alive. Instead, it keeps body fat so it can catch up. Then you just have to stick to losing one or two pounds a week. If you can do so for a year, you can eventually lose between fifty and 100 pounds!

As we have discussed the calculations before, it's time to get to the details. What type of meal should you eat? Which should you be avoiding at all costs?

Let's get off to the positive side. There's plenty of delicious food out there that still lets you hold and lose weight. Don't fall for fad diets that pretend low carbs or no fats will deliver the best result for you. Such diets are only out of your desperation to get income. All foods are required for a healthy physique. You just have to make them work accordingly. Doctors and nutritionists are the best experts to speak with on meal choices. They're giving your money value and they're just looking for your health.

A decent diet should include the right amounts of fats, carbohydrates, and proteins. An average healthy adult requires a fat content of 30 per cent of their calorie intake. So, if you eat 2000 calories a day, you'll get 400 to 600 calories from fat. As 9 calories are contained in 1 gram of fat, the average person will need to eat 44 to 66 grams each day.

The best sources of fat are recipes for nuts, beans, olive and canola oil, avocados, fish oil, and flax seed oil. Weight reducers should note that when it comes from healthy foods, fat really doesn't make you "fat." Fat won't get in your way of losing weight. It'll just add to your health and boost your stamina. As long as you get your fat from the sources mentioned, there's no need to worry.

Carbohydrates are another popular forms of food for fad dieters. It is recommended that you eat 50 per cent of your calorie intake from carbs. The ratio you have to remember: Four calories are one gram of carbohydrates. So someone consuming 2000 calories a day will have to eat a thousand of carbohydrates. Therefore, one has to eat 250 grams of carbohydrates a day. Fruit, vegetables, oatmeal, sweet potatoes, beans, and brown rice are the healthy sources of the carbs. To put it another way, eat complex carbohydrates rather than simple carbs. Simple carbohydrates come from a sugary diet such as white rice, white bread, soda and other highly processed foods.

As for protein, for every kg of your body weight the recommended minimum daily amount is 0.8 grams. Divide the weight by 2.2 then subtract by 0.8 to adjust for this. Since that is merely the minimum, people taking part in workouts should consume more than the calculated amount. To assure your safety you can eat a little more. Chicken, chicken, beef, lean meats, egg / egg whites, nuts, and beans are the best protein options.

Let's go ahead with the meals that you must avoid. Obviously most of those foods are very bad for your well-being. Soft drinks, fast-food, sweets, cookies, pastries and chips are the things not to eat. Besides these, don't eat trans-and saturated fat foods. Stay away from the meals that have elevated levels of sodium and sugar. Generally those meals are where you get your extra calories. You'll drive yourself toward an unhealthy lifestyle aside from the extra pounds.

Now that we've discussed the diet, it's time to talk about exercise. Working out is the best way to have calories burned. It will also increase your strength, flexibility and stamina in addition to weight loss. It will also help you escape heart disease and bone loss over the long run.

For you to participate in 2 types of exercise: aerobic and anaerobic. Aerobic exercise has become more common as cardiovascular workouts. Cardio exercises improve your cardiovascular endurance, performed in moderate to average strength at a lasting rate. Cardio activities include sports such as walking, skating, jogging, swimming, riding, and elliptical machine. The most prescribed exercise in cardiology is one you enjoy, and you are eager to participate in as usual. Those who love walking should do a walk every day. While swimming is perfect for water lovers, bikers can continue with their pastime. The recommended schedule is thirty minutes, in terms of their time. Those still able to carry on above will extend it. The average person is however recommended for the thirty minutes. Do aerobic exercise roughly three to six days a week.

Anaerobic exercise focusses on your muscle and endurance. They usually involve weight training, calisthenics (such as pushups), and the use of resistance machines. Anaerobic workouts are burning you a considerable amount of calories.

Although it isn't as many as cardio workouts, the cardio exercises will improve your stamina. It will produce very good appearances on your body, too. The muscle gain would make you look more toned and sexier. Anaerobic exercises advise speed is between two to four times a week.

There are also some diet legends that everybody should ignore. The first is the misconception of Servings consuming fat and carbohydrates: you fat. Didn't we simply state that fat and carbs are necessary for the health of a person? You need those types of foods to maintain your calories. The next ones are those stupid and pointless one-meal diets. Eating just a little celery or cabbage soup just kills you. Only eating one tiny piece of food won't burn your fat. Your body will simply respond to food shortages and keep your current fat running.

Another myth is that workouts on spot reduction let you lose all your fats. The answer is not to focus on one single area. This is because you focus on your muscles during workouts. Unless fat wraps the muscles, they'll tend to be covered. You'll have to reduce that fat to show off your muscles.

Those products sold in infomercials are the most obvious fallacies. People don't lose their fat by relying on a single product. The same goes for those machines ab. These devices are just yet another example of spot reduction. Any other quick or easy means of reducing weight is simply out to get your money. You have to understand that weight loss requires perseverance and a substantial amount of time.

You should make use of a gym membership if you want to invest cash for your weight loss. The gyms have aerobic and anaerobic exercise machines. It is a powerful motivator, as well. You wouldn't want to spend your money and not take advantage of that membership. You're inspired by the people around you, too. Other means that will help you to reduce weight: digital food scale, treadmill, bike, elliptical machine, weights, tape measurement and a body weight scale.

You need to eat smaller foods more habitually as regards your diet. Eating one to three large meals a day isn't recommended. Instead, break it up into 5 to 6 small meals. Consume the meals every two to three hours. Another way of improving your diet is to prepare your meals. Plan it for the start of the week, and cook it early. This way, the unhealthy meals offered in restaurants or fast-food places don't bpund you. You should also be taking water to your food. Drink this while you eat the meal. The water will make you full quicker and will save you from eating extra calories. Don't eat really quickly. It's going to take the body some time to realize that it is getting full. Gradually grind the food, and don't eat in a rush. When you eat too much, you'll be eating more than your body actually needs.

If you're just starting a routine on weight loss, you have to know it's a long-term activity. You will need to retain the weight by measuring your progress and making the necessary measurements. When you fail to do so, you're going to get that whole weight too fast again. Being safe is a change in lifestyle-a true commitment to the needs of your body.

Myths About Weight Loss.

Do you really know what weight-loss takes? Can you really believe what those statements tell you? Are you confused about what all of those experts tell you? Do you know that 95% of people on conventional diets regain all the weight they've lost and often end up being fatter than when they started? Do you really know what the truth is, and what the speculation is?

Safely, healthily and permanently losing weight isn't as complicated as it might seem. You will finally lose the hideous fat until you know what works and what doesn't and then apply this information properly.

The book is about the most common myths related to weight loss. Understanding them will help to clear up the confusion and help you decide how best to forever lose that weight.

To starve to death is the best way to lose weight.

Losing weight by failing to eat is an absolute no. For that there are three main reasons. The metabolism will be significantly reduced by very low calorie diet or any "fast weight loss" Eating improves metabolism thanks to the energy needed to digest and consume the food. The calories required to digest, consume, transport and metabolize the food we eat will cause our daily caloric expenditure to increase by 10 per cent. Every time we eat, we get a temporary boost to our body's metabolism. So eat little and smaller, more frequent meals and snacks is one way of helping to increase metabolic rates. Skipping meals will cause our metabolic rate to go down until we eat something again.

Reducing the calories significantly lowers our metabolic rate. Our body treats any drastic drop in food intake as an imminent circumstance of starvation and prepares itself to save calories by slowing down our metabolism. The more that we cut our calories drastically, the more that our metabolic rate drops.

Losing weight by dieting alone without exercise depletes our stocks of muscle tissue. Every day, muscle demands a lot more calories to maintain itself. The sooner we lose weight by dieting alone the more we lose muscle tissue and the lower our metabolic rate becomes. Exercise avoids loss of muscle tissue and adds muscle mass and thus increases our metabolic rate.

A Low Fat Diet is Best.

Certain amounts of fats are essential, since the body can not make some fatty acids and must come from the diet. (Fatty acids are actually one of the major components of fat along with cholesterol) Many essential vitamins (A D E K) are only fat-soluble and the fatty acids serve as their carrier.

Certain fatty acids are also essential in cell membrane formation, especially in the nerve tissue.

Patients on a fat-free diet have been shown to develop scaly skin, infertility and have a greater risk of infection.

The different types of fat are yet another source of confusion. We have heard in particular about saturated fat, unsaturated fat, monounsaturated fat and polyunsaturated fat. By going into the chemical variations between each of these fats, it's enough to say good fats and bad fats exist.

The poor fats are saturated fats. They are generally the ones that are solid at room temperature, and tend to be derived from animal sources. That is, butter originates from milk. Too much saturated fat is thought to cause heart disease, diabetes, hypertension and cancers.

Unsaturated fats (both mono & poly) are the good fats, are usually liquid at room temperature and are derived from vegetable sources. So keep an eye on the types of fat in the foods we eat when we look at fats, and stay away from those that are high in saturated fat.

Now that we know what fat is we should eat how much? It's generally accepted that about 30 percent of our calories should come from fat and that no more than 11 percent should come from saturated fat. Therefore, if we take a typical male on 2500 calories, its fat target is not more than 750 calories (or 84 g) from fat. Remember that the maximum allowable amounts are these. Error on the low side of this figure is much better, but DO NOT go below 20 per cent of calories from fat. (For example 500 calories for our male). Note, our diet needs fat.

Weight gain is genetic. You are inheriting that from your parents

Certainly, what we call tendencies may exist, but there is no such thing as a fat gene passed down from generation to generation. What's inherited are attitudes toward food and overall living. When parents are overweight, their food choices will likely be unhealthy, and their lifestyle will likely be unhealthy. Therefore, their children are exposed to that same unhealthy lifestyle from a very early age. We have little chance to stay at a "natural" weight. By following what their parents have done, they have learned to be unhealthy, and will carry this learned behavior with them throughout their lives.

It's not hereditary to be overweight but is another convenient excuse not to try to lose weight. everybody has the power to achieve our weight loss within ourselves.

Fad diets work best to keep weight loss permanent.

Fad diets (Atkins Diet, South Beach Diet, Glycemic Load Diet, etc.) are not the most effective way to lose weight and hold it off. Fad diets also promise a rapid weight loss or advise you to cut off some food from your diet. At first, you might lose weight on one of those diets. But it's hard to follow diets which strictly limit calories or food choices. Most people get tired of them quickly, and recover any weight lost.

Fad diets may be dangerous, as they may not contain all the nutrients that your body needs. In addition, weight loss at a very rapid rate (more than 3 pounds in a week after the first few or couple of weeks) may increase your risk of developing gallstones (gallbladder clusters of solid material that can be painful). Foods that provide less than 800 calories a day may also cause heart rhythm irregularities, which can be fatal.

Research suggests that the best way to lose weight and keep it off is to lose 1/2 pounds to 2 pounds a week by making healthy food choices, eat moderate portions and build physical activity into your daily lives. You can also reduce the risk of developing type 2 diabetes, heart disease and high blood pressure by following healthy eating and physical activity habits.

There are certain types of people who can not lose weight.

We're all born with a fixed amount of fat cells, genetically. Of course some people have more fat cells than others and women have more fat cells than men. The number of cells in fat increases the older we get.

Once it was believed that after adulthood the number of fat cells could not increase; the fat cells could only increase in size. We now know that both size and number of fat cells will actually increase, and that at certain times, as well as under certain circumstances, they are more likely to increase in number.

Existing fat cells grow in size as energy intake exceeds energy expenditure and the excess is deposited in the fat cell. The fat cells of an overweight person can be up to three times larger than those of a person with an ideal body composition.

Fat cells can to increase in number most readily when overweight is gained during the following periods due to overeating and or inactivity:.

- During late infancy and early puberty.
- During pregnancy.
- When extremely large amounts of weight are gained during adulthood.

Except in the case of obesity, the number of fat cells normally stays about the same through adulthood. When the capacity of the existing fat cells is filled, new fat cells can begin to grow to provide extra storage even in adults.

A typical adult who is overweight has some 75 billion fat cells. But however, this number can be as high as 250 to 300 billion in the case of serious obesity!

Because of these facts, some people believe, "Well, I've got more fat cells than others, so I'm never going to lose weight." Many people argue that obesity is hereditary and/or that it is an uphill battle you can't ever overcome once you're obese and your fat cells have multiplied.

To explain your failure it is easy to search for excuses. By looking for seemingly logical and scientific facts and explanations it is easy to justify current circumstances and low future expectations.

Here is the reality.

People who say it can not be done are pessimists or just trying to sell another cure with drugs, remedies or miracles.

Just as some people desperately want to believe in a magic pill or surgical procedure, it always boils down to nutrition and exercise to get a lean body. You can not change the number of fat cells you have (without surgery), but by changing your lifestyle you can shrink every one of them.

The amount of fat cells that you have will certainly influence how hard it will be for you to lose body fat. It is one of the reasons why some people find it harder to lose weight than others as well why some people seem to gain weight more easily than others if their nutrition and exercise programs are not very careful and diligent.

It doesn't mean people can't get lean, though.

The theory of "set point" determines what we shall all weigh.

The set-point theory holds that, like a thermostat, we all have an internal weight control that regulates our metabolic rate up or down as we gain or shed pounds to get our body back to its predetermined mass. Many tests do exist, of course, or we would all be obese or, alternatively, wasting away. Studies show that our metabolism, when we lose weight, actually shifts to a normal rate for that new weight, independent of individual differences. However, it is important that the weight loss is gradual, it is ideal for 1/2 to 2lbs per week. The body doesn't like rapid change as it continues to react to something it doesn't like. For example, our bodies will go into "starvation mode" by rapidly losing weight through diet, where it will slow down our metabolism to preserve our fat reserve: and thus make weight loss very difficult. It will as well tend to make weight gain much more likely when the diet ends because there is so much slowing down in our metabolism.

Nevertheless, people embrace the theory to blame their bodies for their weight-loss failure, rather than their own behaviour. It provides comfort to those who refuse to acknowledge the fact that weight control requires both a physically active and calorie conscious commitment to a lifestyle.

We shouldn't eat late at night, because all that food turns into fat.

The fact is that evening meals don't necessarily make you fat. Too many other variables are involved for making such a large assumption. The primary factor in whether you are gaining or losing fat is not when you are eating but how much. Providing we haven't eaten too many calories for that day when we eat it doesn't really matter.

That doesn't mean meal timing doesn't matter though, It just means that you can eat one of your meals late in the night right before bed and still lose body fat as long as you're in a caloric deficit.

Would be more precise to say that eating large meals late at night before bed, especially high-carbohydrate calorie dense meals, increases the likelihood that you will store some of those calories as fat.

If you plan earlier in the day on eating your calories, and slightly less calories at night, it's probably more beneficial. Research has shown that this can improve fat loss or make it easier to lose fat and that's not the same as saying "eat at night Servings: you fat."

You don't have to exerice to lose weight.

You certainly don't have to exercise to lose weight but if you don't, it's very, very difficult. Most diets fail, because they're too difficult to maintain. Cutting down heavily on calories means we need to deprive ourselves of too many things we enjoy. This leads to cravings leading to cheating leading to failure. It is unhealthy too.

By exercising, we can burn off calories too. In integrating exercise into our regular routine, we're making weight loss more feasible instantly. It can help our weight loss tremendously simply by walking 30 minutes each day at a pace which raises our heart rate enough. Yet the more calories we burn, the more we exercise. In addition, exercise provides us with many other health benefits, such as a healthier heart, lower blood pressure, a greater sense of well-being etc. The benefits are too many to list.

The calorie counting is not essential.

For lose weight, you certainly need to count the calories in one way or another. Most people tend to underestimate their physical activity and their calories. Do not conjecture or attempt to estimate your caloric intake. You just can't be precise enough. There are lots of good computer programs out there that do you most of the work. If your caloric intake (food) is greater than your caloric production (living and exercising) triggers a weight gain, how can you possibly know where you are and what needs to be done?

Missing meals is the best strategy to lose weight.

Studies show that people skipping breakfast and eating less during the day appear to be overweight than people eating a healthy breakfast and eating five to six times a day. This could be because people who skip meals later tend to feel hungry and eat more than they usually would. It is also now generally accepted that people who eat smaller meals, 5 times or 6 times a day, tend to overweight less than others. The feeding cycle itself helps to increase your metabolic rate and, consuming more often, tends to keep your metabolism more active for longer. Note, to keep your caloric intake inside.

Weight loss pills, if you have failed in the past, are the best way to lose weight.

If I said there was a pill that could make you smarter, wealthier or more beautiful, would you believe me. You wouldn't. No. You should probably have laughed at the thought. To assume that a pill could make you lose weight is no longer ludicrous. Many of the so-called weight loss pills on the market have not been tested properly and we are still not sure about the long-term effects of taking them. You're going to read a lot of reviews, praising this or that pill. Ask that to yourself. "Is that review writer trying to sell me something then?" There were no pills yet proven to help weight loss safely and healthily.

High-protein / low-carbohydrate diets represent a healthy way of weight loss.

A high-protein / low-carbohydrate diet does not yet have the long-term health effects. Additionally, it is not a balanced eating plan to get most of your daily calories from high-protein foods like meat, eggs and cheese. You may eat too much cholesterol and fat, which can cause heart disease. You may eat too few fruits, vegetables, and whole grains, which may lead to constipation due to lack of dietary fiber and cause vitamins and minerals to be lacking. It can also make you feel nauseous, exhausted and sluggish following a high-protein / low-carbohydrate diet.

Eating less than 130 grams (520 calories) of carbohydrate per day can cause your body to produce high uric acid levels, which is a risk factor for gout (a painful swelling of the joints) and kidney stones. High-protein / low-carbohydrate diets often have low calories, because food choices are strictly limited, so they can cause weight loss for the short term. But a reduced calorie eating plan that includes recommended amounts of carbohydrate, protein, and fat will also allow weight loss. You will not have to stop eating entire groups of foods, such as whole grains, fruits, and vegetables, by pursuing a healthy eating plan, and lack the key nutrients they provide. You can also find it easier to stick to a diet or eating plan which includes a wider range of foods.

Carbohydrates make you fat.

Carbohydrates won't make you greasy. Calories get you fat. It's often the sugar and the fat in carbohydrates that make you fat. Most carbohydrates are also refined, so you don't get the advantage of feeling full of the fiber contained in unprocessed carbs. Full grain pasta, for example, is more filling and servings: you feel satisfied longer than white pasta, but the same with white bread and brown bread, both have the same calories. What will change the calorie count is how much sauce and butter you put on your pasta. What you want to do is eat a small amount of carbs.

You will lose weight on a particular part of your body.

It is absolutely impossible to lose weight from just a specific part of your body, physically. You can't control where your body takes off fat. Any machine or particular exercise that claims to specifically lose stomach fat or thigh fat is lying. Certainly, a particular exercise in that group of muscles being trained will improve muscle tone, giving the illusion that fat is being lost.

In a predetermined order, fat will just vanish from your body.

Don't weigh yourself.

That you should not get on a scale when trying to lose weight is another myth. It's a good motivational tool to regularly check your weight, say once a week. It's an easy way to assess your progress and change your diet accordingly. It's a bad idea to just use scales, though. Use your eyes to track changes in your body. Make use of measuring tape to keep track of both inches of tummy and thigh.

What you must keep in mind, however, is that basically what you are trying to do is lose fat and not just weight. It is harder to measure fat loss but it is a far better indicator of your success. Assessment of body fat is best done by a doctor and can be done in most of the local gyms or health clubs. There's also a wide range of freely available tools which can give you a fairly precise measurement.

Keys To Change Your Diet To A Successful Weight Loss Over The Long Term.

Do you want to drop pounds? Have you only followed the latest fad diet plan to get back to your old ways and get all the weight back? Think you are the only one that doesn't have the power of will to lose weight? The reality isn't that you are alone. Most people taking on a diet have no long-term success! Why? Because they are choosing a diet program that is unrealistic to their existing habits and is not life-sustainable.

The Cabbage Soup Diet.

I'm just using the cabbage soup diet as an example of something impractical and forever unsustainable. The diet plan had been all the rage at one time. But like all the fads it came and went and left many people frustrated in its wake as they gained all their weight back and maybe some extra. Why? Because you won't have a bowl of cabbage breakfast soup for the rest of your life, lunch and dinner everyday! Cabbage soup is good and nutritious but you'll grow bored of it quickly and start hating it. For one time during the week would have been a good meal is now a bad memory and you will never place your lips on it again.

Secrets to a Long Term Weight Loss!

You must develop habits that can be incorporated into your lifestyle to be successful in weight loss over the long term, and lead you to proper weight management. You have to set up yourself for success by developing a routine around something you already do. You are sleeping, you are drinking, you are getting angry and disappointed and you like to be praised. Those keys will help you develop a pattern around each of those things when linking it to weight loss over the long term.

Sleep!

You sleep and let us see how your weight is influenced by this. We'll start by giving you some recorded sleep research:

· Columbia University Medical Center (CUMC) Scientists found that people who logged five hours of sleep a night were 60 percent more likely than those who slept seven to nine hours. They found that sleep deprivation alters leptin and gherilin levels, which are hormones that regulate appetite, leading to hunger.

· The Obesity Reviews publication posted an article claiming that the more hours you are up, the more you are going to eat. They estimated that an increase in sleep of one hour would reduce caloric intake by 6 per cent or an average of 120 calories.

· Evidence from the American Medical Association Journal has indicated that sleep loss raises appetite while reducing body metabolism.

As you can see from all three of these, lack of sleep is not a winning weight management or weight loss combination but is a weight gain recipe. The key to sleep is getting your rest properly. When you sleep for 5 to 6 hours, you need to start making changes to increase your sleep time to at least 7 hrs of sleep. Perhaps it cuts off the late-night news or television show. Use that time by adding it to your sleep time to recover from your day.

We also help you manage your weight loss and weight loss, proper sleep will help you with some other health problems that could affect your overall health and wellness. A research from the Archives of Internal Medicine found that women who only slept five hrs a night were 2 and 1/2 times more likely to have diabetes than men who slept seven to eight hours a day. Columbia University research has found that women who slept for less than six hours each night have increased their risk of developing high blood pressure by 70 percent over those who slept for seven to eight hours. And, Mount Sinai School of Medicine study has shown that sleep deprivation reduces the immune system, rendering you more susceptible to infection. As you can see, developing the habit of getting your proper rest will be good for your weight loss program and overall health over the long term.

Water!

You drink so let us see how your weight is affected by what you drink. Let's continue with what we know is true:

· The average regular pop of 12 oz can contains 155 calories and 9 teaspoons of sugar. The American average consumes 54 gallons of soda per annum. That is equivalent to 1.5 cans or 230 calories per day all of which are sugar-derived. A pound of fat has 3,500 calories in it. The average American might see a weight gain of 1 lb every 14-15 days from regular pop consumption.

· Many scientific studies have shown that empty soft drink calories are directly linked to weight gain, which in turn becomes a primary risk factor for type 2 diabetes.

· If you think the answer is going to a diet soda, think again. There are numerous studies that link weight gain to diet pop consumption so you haven't satisfied thirst or hunger even if you've reduced your caloric intake. This is causing people to overeat.

· The phenomenon of "Super-Size Me" has produced a sizeable population. The dangers of smoking cigarettes have now been overtaken by obesity and its associated health effects.

Interestingly, experts estimate that 75 per cent of Americans are slightly dehydrated with all we drink. Your body must replace 2 quarts - 3 quarts of water every day; more than 1/2 gallon or more. If the fluid we eat is loaded with sugars and other chemicals, then the liver and body need that water to help detoxify the system. The water can not go to the rest of the cells of the body causing them a mild dehydration that affects the levels of metabolism and energy.

You need water which is pure and odourless. Water does not contain calories, artificial sweeteners or colorings, and is fat-free, cholesterol-free, low in sodium and not acidic. Water is an important part of weight loss and weight management. Most find water to be the most significant factor in fat loss because of its effect on your overall metabolism and helping your body metabolize stored fat. Because water has no calories, without weight gain, you can drink as much as you want, and it Servings: as an appetite suppressant.

Work to cultivate the habit to bring purer water into your body. I managed to find a fantastic Green Fusion product. It is a powder that I add to my water and without shopping and preparing it gives me all the nutritional value of an organic plant-based program. Or, add a limon or a wedge of lime to your water. You may initially find yourself going to the bathroom more frequently but your body will adjust.

Speak of your visits to the toilet as part of your walking routine because it will be good for your weight loss over thc long term. Additionally, proper hydration reduces joint and muscle soreness, reduces back pain, enhances energy and muscle tone, and helps eliminate mental confusion and disorientation.

Anger and Disappointment!

You're getting angry and disappointed so let us see how your emotions affect your weight:

· Researchers at Leeds University have monitored the 422 employees ' behaviors. Researchers noticed that depressed people tended to eat fewer vegetables and snacked on more fattening foods throughout the day instead. When under stress the body produces the hormone cortisol, says Daryl O'Connor, Ph.D., the study's author. Cortisol causes high calorie food cravings.

· Pennsylvania State University researchers looked into the effects of loud noise on feeding. Those who couldn't shut off the noise later consumed twice as many calories as those who could.

· Cynthia Power's research found that your emotions govern what you're snack on. You will usually prefer crunchy foods like chips when you're angry or frustrated, because chewing is a physical release for the emotion. If you're sad, choose a snack that will fill you up like cake, popcorn or pasta. If you're down, then the food of choice is usually sweet, fluffy foods such as chocolate and ice cream as the sugar helps boost your energy and mood.

You will start stressing your life just by the morning commute to work. Add a noisy, busy office environment to that and you're prepared for some serious snacking. You may be a stay-at-home mom with a noisy preschool setting. With the tension of raising the kids and keeping the home from looking like a disaster zone, the nap time is snack time. How do you transfer those emotions that trigger a healthy habit of eating that will separate real hunger from emotional hunger?

The majority of people carry a planner every day. So, make it a habit of carrying a men's journal and a women's diary with your daily planner. (They are both the same but it's easier for men to look at it as a newspaper.) When you feel particularly stressed, take six minutes and enter your newspaper. People will think that you just add an important meeting to your everyday planner. And, you are, in a way. You make a rendezvous to release your emotions which is good personal therapy. If you're still hungry after the six minutes, then go ahead and get a nice little snack to relieve your appetite. Most people find that, when they complete their journal entry, they don't need to eat.

Reward Yourself!

The one overriding characteristic of most diets is denial which is a negative approach rather than a constructive weight management approach. Is there someone who wouldn't like a reward? We just love to receive reward. We lead our rewarding lives. It helps to tame the tension by building rewards into your programme.

· Most experts suggest you get ten percent of your calories from "fun foods." If you're on a diet of 1500 calories, that's 150 calories.

· According to studies from the University of Cincinnati, a small amount of sugar helps your body cope with stress because it can minimize the development of glucocorticoid, a stress hormone related to the accumulation of fat in your abdomen.

· Experts recommend selecting a snack that also contains protein since protein will help slow sugar release into the body. If you can combine that with fiber, better still.

Increase rewards into your programme. If you need a daily reward then build in your program a favorite snack if it meets the criteria of having some protein to offset the sugar; the higher the protein and the better the sugar. Throw it a little fiber and that Servings: much better your everyday reward.

You may want to reward yourself for the weekend, or there's a special event coming up. Bank your daily rewards on weekends for that one day, or for that special event. You did not gain your weight in a day but made those decisions over days, weeks and years. It's important to let yourself have permission to reward yourself. If you've banked your 150 calorie average incentive then you've got 900 calories to reward yourself on that weekend day. Enjoy them, and then return the next day to work on the target of weight loss or weight management.

Easy and Delicious SirtFood Recipes.

If you're going to try the Sirtfood Diet, we're here to give you a helping hand, with delicious recipes.

The Sirtfood Juice.

A good way to get started is with The Sirtfood Juice – so we've thrown this in the recipe to start you off as an extra bonus.

Sirtfood Green Juice

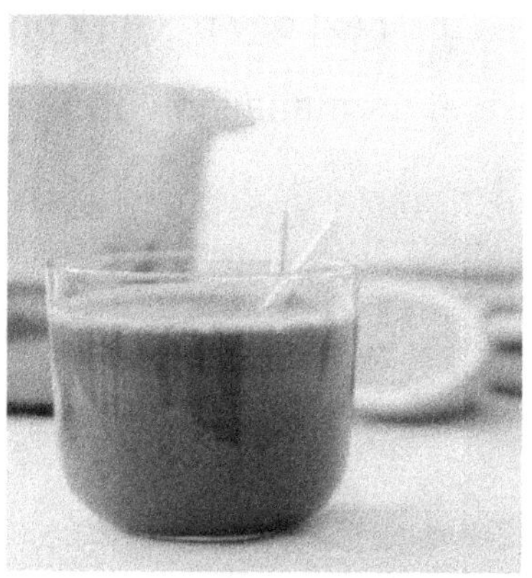

Servings: 1

Ingredients:

- a very small handful flat-leaf parsley (5g)
- a very small handful lovage leaves (5g) (optional)
- 2–3 large stalks green celery (150g) , including its leaves
- 2 large handfuls (75g) kale
- a large handful (30g) rocket
- ½ medium green apple
- juice of ½ lemon
- ½ level teasp matcha green tea

Instructions:

- Mix together the greens (kale, rocket, parsley and lovage, if used), then sauté them. We think juicers can really vary in their efficiency when juicing leafy vegetables and before going on to the other ingredients, you may need to re-juice the remains. The goal is to finish off the greens with around 50ml of juice.

- Now you can peel the lemon and also bring it through the juicer, but we find it much easier to actually by hand squeeze the lemon in the juice. You need to have about 250ml of juice in total by this point, maybe a little bit more.

It's only when the juice is made and ready to serve that you add the green tea matcha.

- In a glass, pour a small amount of juice, then add the matcha, and stir vigorously with a fork or teaspoon. At day's first two drinks, we only use matcha, because it contains moderate amounts of caffeine (the same content as a normal tea cup). if drunk late, After dissolution of the matcha add the rest of the juice, it may keep them awake for people not used to it.

- Give it a stir finish, then your juice is ready to drink. Free to top up with plain water, as you like.

Nutrition Info

90. Cal. 91%. 20g. Carbs. 0%. Fat. 9%. 2g. Protein.

Shredded Chicken Bowl

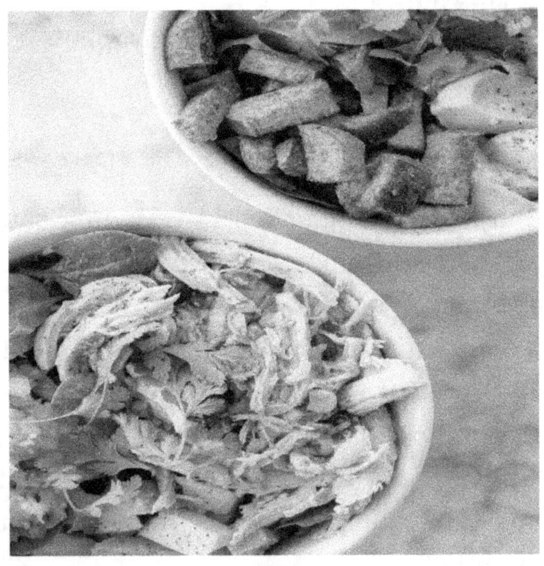

Prep Time:10 min.
Cook Time:35 min.
Total Time:45 min.
Serving 3-5

Ingredients:

- 1 jar of roasted tomato salsa or corn salsa/black bean
- 2-3 cups organic spinach (for your base)
- 1/2 cup cilantro
- Lime
- Coconut aminos

- 2 organic chicken breasts
- 1 jar of salsa verde
- 2 ripe avocados
- 1/4-1/2 cup jalapeño sauerkraut

Instructions

- Put/place the chicken breasts in a saucepan with one full salsa verde jar and half a roasted tomato jar or black bean / corn salsa.
- Cover and cook for 25 minutes on medium to low heat, or until chicken is cooked through.
- When cooked through, remove the chicken and shred it with two forks, then put it back in the pot then heat for another 5 minutes-10 minutes.
- Place your spinach base and drizzle with the coconut aminos in your serving bowls.
- Add the shredded, cooked chicken into the bowl. (Vegetarian Sub Sweet Potatoes.) 6. For each bowl, add half a cut ripe avocado.
- Add 2 spoonfuls of sauerkraut per bowl.
- On each bowl, squeeze half a lime, and sprinkle with cilantro.

Nutrition Info

Calories 520 (2176 kJ)
Cholesterol 85 mg

28%
Sodium 1200 mg
50%
Total Carbohydrate 54 g
18%
Dietary Fiber 9 g

Buckwheat and Nut Loaf

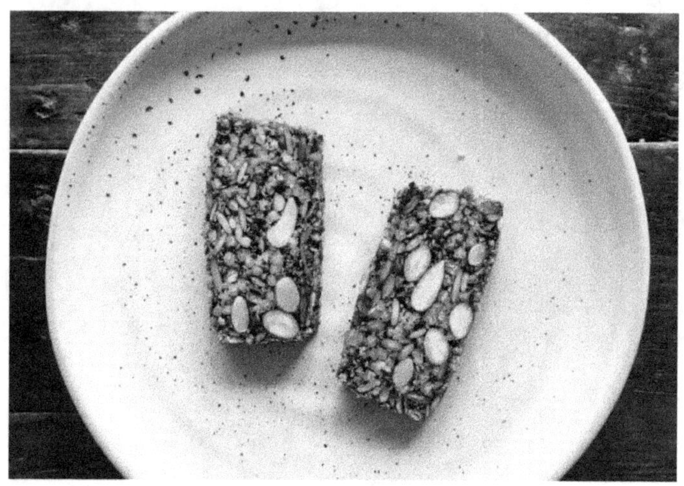

Servings: 4

Ingredients

- 2 tbsp olive oil
- 225g/8oz mushrooms
- 2-3 carrots, finely diced
- 225g/8oz buckwheat
- 2-3 tbsp fresh herbs, finely chopped eg: marjoram, oregano, thyme, parsley
- 225g/8oz nuts eg: almonds, hazelnuts, walnuts
- 2 eggs, beaten
- Salt and pepper

Instructions

- Place the buckwheat in a pan with 350ml/1.5 cup pan of water and a pinch of salt. Take to boil. Cover and cook with the lid until all the water is absorbed-about 10-15 minutes.
- Meanwhile, sauté the olive oil into the mushrooms and carrots until tender.
- Blitz the food processor's nuts, until well chopped.
- Stir in the eggs and combine the vegetables, cooked buckwheat, herbs and chopped nuts. If you are using tahini instead of eggs mix this with some water before stirring it into the buckwheat to create a thick pouring consistency.
- Mix with pepper and salt.
- Transfer to a oiled or lined loaf tin and bake for 30 minutes in the oven at gas mark 5/190C until set and just brown on top.

Sweet Potato and Salmon Patties

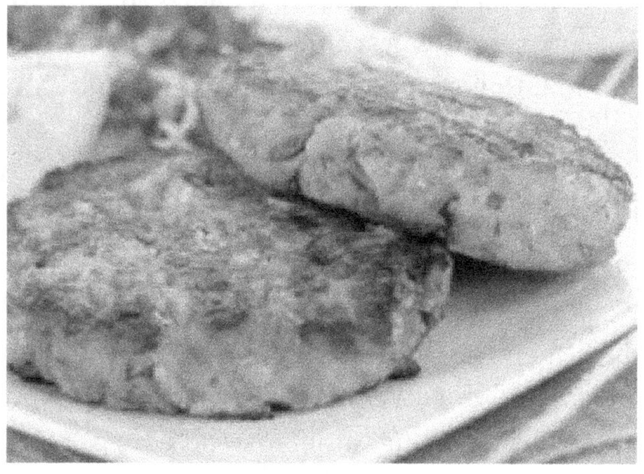

Servings: 4

Ingredients

- Rice flour or buckwheat flour
- 225g/8oz wild salmon, cooked or tinned
- 225g/8oz sweet potato cooked and mashed
- Herb salt and pepper to taste

Instructions

- Preheat the oven upto 160C / gas mark 3.
- Mix the sweet potato, salmon, herbal salt and pepper together. Take a small size handful of the mixture and shape it into a ball. Flatten

into a shape of burger then dip into the flour on each side. Place it on a lined baking tray. Repeat until the blend is used up.

- Bake only turning once for 20 minutes. Serve with a sizeable green salad.

Nutrition Info

116 Cal, 13g Carbs, 2g Fat, 9g Protein

Trout with Roasted Vegetables

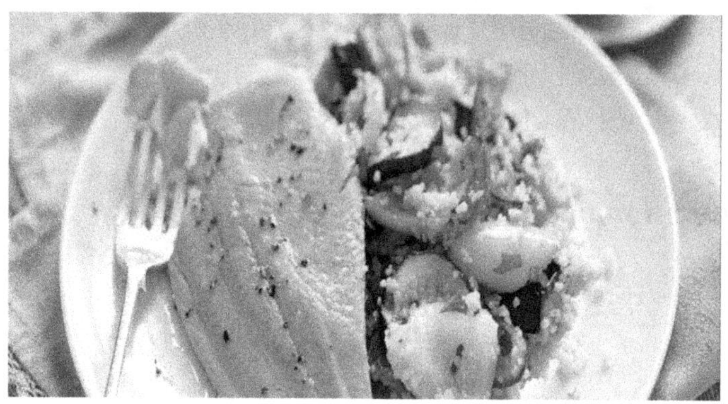

Servings: 2

Ingredients

- 2 turnips, peeled and cut into segments
- Olive oil
- Dried dill
- Juice of 1 lemon
- 2 carrots, cut into batons
- 2 parsnips, peeled and cut into wedges
- Tamari
- 1 trout fillet per person

Instructions

- Put the sliced vegetables into a baking tray. Sprinkle with a dash of tamari and olive oil. Set on gas mark 7 in the oven. Take the vegetables out of the oven after 25 minutes, and stir well.

- Put the fish over it. Sprinkle with the dill and lemon juice. Cover with foil, and go back to the oven.
- Turn down the oven to gas mark 5/190C/375F and cook till the fish is cooked through for 20 minutes.

Butterbean and Vegetable Korma

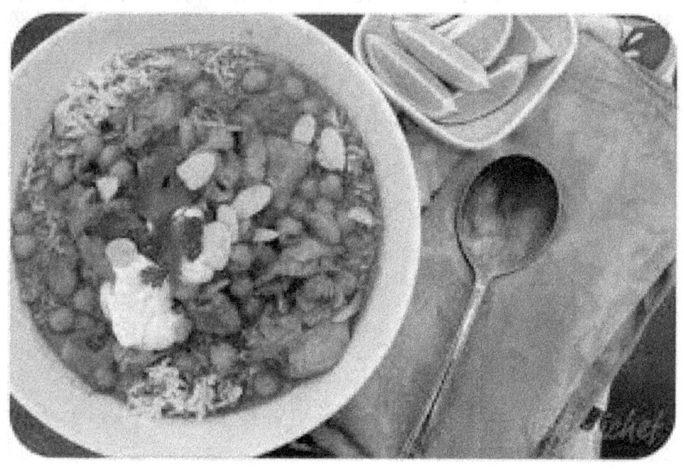

Servings: 4

Ingredients

- 1 clove of garlic, finely chopped
- 1-2 tbsp curry powder
- 3 sweet potatoes, peeled & chopped into large chunks
- 2 cans of butterbeans
- 50-100g/2-4ounce creamed coconut
- 3 tbsp coconut oil or olive oil
- 1 large onion, finely chopped
- 200g/7ounce green beans, cut into 2 cm lengths
- 1 cauliflower, cut into florets

- 2 tsp root ginger, finely chopped
- 1 tbsp chopped coriander

Instructions

- In a large pan/saucepan heat up the oil and add the onion. Cook the onions until they are soft
- Add the garlic & ginger to the onions, and cook for a few minutes.
- Adding the green beans, cauliflower and sweet potatoes into the curry powder and mix well to cover in the spices.
- Add butter beans drained and rinsed, and enough hot water to cover the ingredients.
- Cook for 20 minutes -30 minutes, or until cooked through the vegetables.
- Transfer some liquid from the saucepan to the bowl and dissolve the coconut cream inside. Remove this to the saucepan and cook for several minutes.
- Just before you serve, sprinkle over the fresh coriander.

Nutrition Info

Calories: 218kcal, Fat: 7.73g, Carbs: 26.16g, Prot: 11.76g

Baked salmon with stir fried vegetables

Servings: 2

Ingredients

- Grated zest and juice of 1 lemon
- 1 teasp toasted sesame oil
- 2 teasp olive oil
- 2 carrots, cut into matchsticks
- Bunch of kale, chopped
- 2 teasp of root ginger, grated
- 2 wild salmon fillets
- 1 tin of water chestnuts, drained, rinsed & chopped

Instructions

- Mix the lemon juice and ginger and zest together. Place the salmon in a shallow, oven proof dish and pour over the lemon ginger mixture. Cover with foil and leave for 30-60 minutes to marinate.
- Bake the salmon on gas mark 5/190C in the oven for 15 minutes while cooking heat up a wok or frying pan then add the toasted sesame oil and olive oil. Add the vegetables,

and cook, stirring constantly for a few minutes.

- Once the salmon are cooked spoon some of the salmon marinade onto the vegetables and cook for a few more minutes.
- Serve the vegetables onto a plate and top with salmon.

Lemon paprika chicken with vegetables

Servings: 2

Ingredients

- 2 carrots, chopped
- 2 bay leaves
- Salt and pepper
- Juice of 1 lemon
- ½ a celeriac, peeled and chopped
- 3 turnips, peeled and chopped
- 300g of chicken wings
- 3 tbsp olive oil
- 2 tbsp paprika
- 1 pint of hot stock
- Sprigs of rosemary and thyme
- Large bunch of kale, chopped

Instructions

- Heat the oil with a tight fitting lid inside a large saucepan. Add the carrots, paprika, celeriac, chicken and turnip wings to the saucepan and cook for a few minutes.
- Stir in the pan the stock, spices, salt, pepper and lemon juice and bring to the boil.

- Turn the heat down, cover it with a lid and gently simmer for 40 minutes.
- Add the kale and cook until the kale and the chicken are both cooked for a few more minutes.

Nutrition Info

Calories 154.0
Total Fat 2.2 g
Saturated Fat 0.7 g
Cholesterol 67.7 mg
Dietary Fiber 0.9 g
Sugars 2.6 g
Protein

Sirtfood Bites

Servings: 15 - 20 BITES

Ingredients:

- 1 oz (30g) dark chocolate (85 percent cocoa solids), broken into pieces; or 1/4 cup cocoa nibs
- 1 cup (120g) walnuts
- the scraped 1 vanilla pod seeds or 1 teaspoon vanilla extract
- 1 to 2 tablespoons water
- 9 ounces (250g) Medjool dates, pitted
- 1 tablespoon cocoa powder
- 1 tablespoon ground turmeric
- 1 tablespoon extra virgin olive oil

Instructions

- Place the chocolate and walnuts in a food processor and process them until the powder is perfect.
- Add all the remaining ingredients except water and mix until the mixture forms a ball. Depending on the consistency of the mixture, you may or may not have to apply the water- you don't want it to be too messy.

- Form the mixture into bite-size balls using your hands and cool in an airtight container for at least 1 hour before eating them.
- In some more cocoa or dried coconut you could roll some of the balls to achieve a different finish, if you like. You can keep it in your fridge for up to 1 week.

Raw carrot and almond loaf

Servings: 4

Ingredients

- ½ cup of almonds
- Fresh parsley, finely chopped
- 6-8 carrots, grated
- Juice of ½ a lemon
- 4 tbsp of tahini

Instructions

- With the S blade, place the grated carrots in a food processor.
- Whizz over the carrots with the lemon juice until well homogenized. Put them in a saucepan.
- Then whizz up in the food processor until the almonds are ground down.
- Adding the carrot mixture to the almonds, and mix with the chopped parsley and tahini.
- Pack this into a tin loaf and cut it into slices for serving.

Savoury Seed Truffles

Servings: 2

Ingredients

- Pinch of cayenne pepper
- Juice of half a lemon
- 60g/2oz pumpkin seeds
- 60g/2oz sunflower seeds
- 2 tbsp tahini
- A handful of coriander leaves
- Salt and pepper

Instructions

- Put the seeds with the S blade in a food processor, and grind thoroughly.
- Stir in the tahini, cayenne, lemon juice, leaves of coriander, and salt and pepper.
- Process until the mixture stays in place adding as appropriate small amounts of water.
- Take away the blade from the food processor and mold the mixture into balls filled with walnuts.

Almond Butter and Alfalfa Wraps

Servings: 4

Ingredients

- 4 tbsp of almond nut butter
- Juice of 1 lemon
- 2-3 carrots – grated
- 3 radishes, finely sliced
- 1 cup of alfalfa sprouts
- Salt and pepper
- Lettuce leaves or nori sheets

Instructions

- Combine the almond butter with most of the lemon juice and enough water to make the consistency creamy.
- Mix the grated carrot, the alfalfa sprouts in a bowl. Sprinkle with the remaining lemon juice, and add salt and pepper to season.
- Spread the almond buttered lettuce leaves or nori sheets, and top with the mixture of carrots and sprouts. Roll up immediately, and feed!

Courgette Tortilla

Servings: 2

Ingredients

- 4 eggs, beaten
- A pinch of salt and pepper
- 2 tbsp coconut oil or butter
- 1 courgettes, sliced
- Freshly chopped chives or parsley

Instructions

- Heat the butter/oil in a heavy bottomed frying pan then add the courgettes. Cook until soft, be stirring occasionally.
- Mix the pepper, salt, and herbs in with the beaten eggs then add to the pan
- Cook till the egg is nearly cooked through. Complete the cooking by placing the pan under the medium grill. Serve with a large green salad.

Asian king prawn stir-fry with buckwheat noodles

Servings: 1

Ingredients:

- 150g shelled raw king prawns, deveined
- 1 tsp finely chopped fresh ginger
- 20g red onions, sliced
- 2 teasp tamari (you can use soy sauce if you are not avoiding gluten)
- 2 teasp extra virgin olive oil
- 50g kale, roughly chopped
- 100ml chicken stock
- 5g lovage or celery leaves
- 75g soba (buckwheat noodles)
- 1 garlic clove, finely chopped
- 1 bird's eye chilli, finely chopped
- 40g celery, trimmed and sliced
- 75g green beans, chopped

Instructions:

- Heat up a saucepan over high heat, then cook the prawns for 2–3 minutes in 1 teaspoon tamari and 1 teaspoon oil. Put the prawns onto a plate. Wipe the pan out with paper from the kitchen, as you will be using it again.

- Cook the noodles 5–8 minutes in boiling water, or as indicated on the packet. Drain and set aside.
- Meanwhile, over medium - high heat, fry the garlic, chilli and ginger, red onion, celery, beans and kale in the remaining oil for 2 minutes–3 minutes. Adding the stock and bring to the boil, then cook for one or two minutes until the vegetables are cooked but crunchy.
- Add the prawns, noodles and leaves of lovage / celery to the pan, bring back to the boil, then remove the heat and serve.

Polenta Bake

Servings: 4-6

Ingredients

- 2 tsp dried oregano
- 1 cup of sun-dried tomatoes, chopped
- 3 eggs, separated
- 850ml/1.5 pints of water
- 1 tsp rock salt or sea salt
- 300g/10oz red Leicester cheese ar cheddar, grated (optional)
- 200g/7oz coarse yellow polenta
- 1-2 tbsp butter or olive oil
- Freshly ground black pepper

Instructions

- Inside the large saucepan, bring the water to boil with the salt to cook the polenta.
- Slowly pour in the stirring polenta the whole time. Add the sun-dried tomatoes and the oregano.
- Cook on low heat, as long as the polenta packet instructions say. It could be from 3 minutes to 40 minutes at any location.

Regularly stir up to prevent clumping and sticking.

- While the polenta cooks whip the whites of the eggs until they form stiff peaks.
- When the polenta is cooked, turn off the heat and stir the egg yolks and black pepper in 1-2 tbsp of butter or olive oil along with 2/3 of the cheese, if used. Add extra salt if needed.
- Carefully fold the egg whites into the polenta blend.
- Transfer the mixture to a proof dish oiled with oven. Spread and the top smooth.
- Sprinkle over the remaining grated cheese.
- Bake for 40-50 minutes at gas mark 4/180C/350F, until set and start to brown.

Buckwheat Pancakes

Servings: 4

Ingredients

- 1 free range egg, beaten
- Butter, olive oil/coconut oil for frying
- 1 cup of natural soya yoghurt
- 110g/4oz buckwheat flour
- ½ tsp of salt
- 1 cup of water

Instructions

- Inside a mixing bowl, combine flour and salt, and make a well in the centre.
- Combine the egg, yogurt, and water in the jug and gradually beat this into the flour until a smooth batter is in place. Let it to rest for an hour or longer.
- In a frying pan, heat some oil and drop tablespoons of the batter into the pan.
- Cook for a few minutes before turning gently, until the underside begins to brown. Cook until done, for a few more minutes.
- Continue on until all the batter has been used.

Pea, Miso and Mint Soup

Servings: 2

Ingredients

- 2 tbsp olive oil
- 1 red onion (optional), finely chopped
- Salt and pepper
- 300g/10oz of frozen peas
- 2 tbsp fresh mint, chopped
- 4 tablesp natural yoghurt or soya yoghurt (optional)
- 1 tsp miso

Instructions

- Inside a saucepan heat the oil, and add the onion. Cook until tender.
- Add the frozen peas and boiling water to 700ml.
- Bring to boil for a few minutes and simmer.
- Add the mint, salt, miso, and pepper and mix until smooth, using a hand blender.
- If using, serve in bowls and mix in yoghurt.

Buckwheat Kasha with Mushrooms and Onions

Buckwheat Kasha with Sauteed Mushrooms, Peas and Onions, Drizzled with truffle oil for a touch of decadence. This naturally gluten-free side dish is finished in 20 minutes, and owing to the nutrients in the buckwheat groats it is super healthy.

Prep Time5 mins
Cook Time15 mins
Total Time20 mins
Servings: 4

Ingredients

- 1 cp uncooked buckwheat
- 2 cps vegetable or chicken broth for cooking the buckwheat (or use water)
- 10 ounce baby bella mushrooms, cleaned and sliced or quartered
- 1 cup frozen or fresh peas (no need to thaw if using frozen)
- 3 tablespoons chopped parsley leaves
- 2 tablespoons olive oil
- 1 yellow onion, thinly sliced
- 1 tablespoon truffle-infused olive oil
- Salt & pepper to taste

- In a medium saucepan, combine uncooked buckwheat and vegetable broth (or water). Season with a pinch of salt and pepper, when sodium-free broth. Bring to a boil and cover then bring down heat. Cook for about 10 minutes, or tender until buckwheat. When liquid still exists, rinse off extra liquid. While cooking the buckwheat, prepare the rest of the platter.

- Heat 2 tblespns of olive oil over medium heat in a large skillet, and add the sliced onion. Saute for 5 mins, or until the onion begins softening and turning golden brown. Remove the mushrooms, and saute in the skillet for 5 minutes or until the mushrooms begin to sweat.

- When the mushrooms start releasing juices, add the frozen (or fresh) peas and saute until they are heated through for 3 minutes. Season with salt for tasting, and freshly ground pepper.

- Add the cooked buckwheat and the chopped parsley to the skillet and combine all the flavors well over medium heat. Turn off the heat, and sprinkle with truffle oil. Taste it to see if there's more salt to add. Serving warm.

Nutrition Info

Calories 294 Calories from Fat 63
Fat 7g11%
Sodium 5mg0%
Potassium 357mg10%
Carbohydrates 5g2%
Sugar 2g2%
Protein 2g

Sirt Muesli

Just mix the dry ingredients and place them in an airtight container If you want to do this in bulk or have it prepared the night before. In the next day all you need to do is add the strawberries and yoghurt and it's ready to go.

Servings: 1

Ingredients:

- 15g walnuts, chopped
- 10g cocoa nibs
- 15g coconut flakes or desiccated coconut
- 100g strawberries, hulled and chopped
- 20g buckwheat flakes
- 40g Medjool dates, pitted then chopped
- 100g plain Greek yoghurt
- 10g buckwheat puffs

Instructions:

- Combine and mix all the above ingredients together (leave out the strawberries and yoghurt if not immediately served).

Buckwheat Noodle and Green Bean Soup

Servings: 4

Ingredients

- 2 carrots, cut into thin strips
- 1 litre of boiling water
- 400g buckwheat noodles
- 1 tbsp tamari soy sauce
- 2 tbsp olive oil
- 1 tsp toasted sesame oil
- 1 tsp ginger root, finely sliced
- 2 spring onions, finely sliced
- 1 tbsp rice wine (optional)
- 125g/4oz frozen edamame beans
- Fresh coriander, finely chopped
- Salt and pepper

Instructions

- Heat the olive then sesame oil in a wok or large saucepan. Stir in the spring onions, ginger root, and carrots then cook for a few minutes.
- Pour a liter of boiling water over it. When it's bubbling add the noodles, edamame beans, tamari, & rice wine.
- Cook until the vegetables & noodles are just cooked.
- Garnish with leaves of coriander and, if desired, season with salt and pepper.

Sirtfood Diet's smoked salmon omelette

Try this fast and easy Sirtfood dish full of flavour and goodness

Servings: 1
Prep Time: 0 hours 5 mins
Cook Time: 0 hours 0 mins
Total Time: 0 hours 5 mins

Ingredients

- 2 Medium eggs
- 100 g Smoked salmon, sliced
- 1/2 tsp. Capers
- 10 g Rocket, chopped
- 1 tsp. Parsley, chopped
- 1 tsp. Extra virgin olive oil

Instructions

- Crack the eggs and whisk well in a bowl. Add the salmon, capers, parsley and rocket.
- In a non-stick frying pan, heat up the olive oil until hot but not smoking. Add the egg mixture and move the mixture around the pan, using a spatula or fish slice, until it is even. Reduce heat, and let cook through the omelet. Slide the spatula around edges and roll the omelet up or fold in half to serve.

Chicken breast with kale,red onions, a tomato and chilli salsa

Servings: 1

Ingredients:

- juice of 1/4 lemon
- 1 tablespoon extra virgin olive oil
- 3/4 cup (50g) kale, chopped
- 1/8 cup (20g) red onion, sliced
- 1/4 pound skinless, boneless chicken breast
- 2 tsps ground turmeric
- 1 teaspoon chopped fresh ginger
- 1/3 cup (50g) buckwheat

FOR THE SALSA

- 1 medium tomato (130g)
- 2 tablespoons (5g) parsley, finely chopped
- juice of 1/4 lemon
- 1 Thai chili, finely chopped
- 1 tablespoon capers, finely chopped

Instructions:

- Remove the eye from the tomato to make the salsa, and chop it very fine, taking care to keep the liquid as much as possible. Mix/combine with the chilli, capers, lemon juice and parsley. You might put it all in a blender but the end result is a bit different.

- Oven heat to 220oC / gas 7. Marinate the chicken breast with the turmeric, lemon juice and a little oil in 1 teaspoon. Heat an ovenproof frying pan until dry, then add the marinated chicken and cook on each side for about a min or so until pale golden, then move to the oven (place on a baking tray if your pan is not ovenproof) for 8 minutes-10 minutes or until cooked through. And remove from the oven, cover with foil and leave to rest before serving for 5 minutes.

- Meanwhile, boil the kale for 5 minutes in a steamer. In a little oil, fry the red onions and ginger until soft but not colored, then add the cooked kale & fry for another minute. Fry the buckwheat with the remaining turmeric teaspoon in accordance with the packet instructions. Serve with chicken, tomatoes, and salsa.

Cauliflower and Chickpea Masala

This easy, super creamy, and heavily spiced Cauliflower and Masala Chickpea will be your new favorite weekend dinner! So much sugar, so little commitment.

Prep Time: 10 mins
Cook Time: 30 mins
Total Time: 40 mins

Ingredients

Masala Spice Mix

- 2 Tbsp garam masala
- 1/2 tsp cumin
- 1/2 tsp turmeric
- 1/2 tsp smoked paprika
- 1/4 tsp cayenne
- 1/2 tsp salt
- Freshly Cracked Pepper

Skillet Ingredients

- 1 yellow onion
- 3 cloves garlic
- 1/2 Tbsp grated fresh ginger

- 2 Tbsp olive oil
- 12 oz. frozen cauliflower florets
- 1 15oz. can chickpeas, drained
- 1 15oz. can tomato sauce
- 1/4 cup water
- 1/3 cup heavy cream
- salt to taste

Instructions

- In a small bowl, add the spices (turmeric, garam masala, cumin,smoked paprika, salt, cayenne, and pepper) for the masala spice mix.
- Dice the onion finely, slim the garlic and grind the ginger. Along with the olive oil, add all three to a large skillet and Saute over medium heat until soft and translucent onions (around 3 mins). Add the spice mixture and continue sautéing for another minute.
- Adding the frozen cauliflower florets with the aromatics and spices to the skillet and continue sautéing for about 5 minutes, or until the cauliflower has thawed through and is completely covered in spices.
- Fill the skillet with the drained chickpeas, tomato sauce and 1/4 cup water. Remove to mix, then allow them to simmer for about 15 minutes over medium-low heat, stirring

occasionally. This will help to mellow the tomato sauce acidity and encourage the spices to blend together. If the mixture gets too dry as it simmers, then add a few more spoonfuls of water.

- Switch/turn off the heat and stir in the heavy cream after the sauce has simmered for 15 minutes. Give a taste to the masala, and add salt as needed. Serve in a bowl for dipping, either over rice or with a piece of bread.

Nutrition Info

Calories: 306.9kcal · Protein: 9.58g · Fat: 16.48g · Carbohydrates: 33.3g · Sodium: 1153.2mg · Fiber: 10.45g

Sirtfood bites

(Servings: 15-20 bites)

Ingredients:

- 250g Medjool dates, pitted
- 1 tbsp cocoa powder
- 1 tbsp ground turmeric
- 120g walnuts
- 1 tbsp extra virgin olive oil
- 30g dark chocolate (85% cocoa solids), broken into pieces; or cocoa nibs
- the scraped 1 vanilla pod seeds or 1 teasp vanilla extract
- 1–2 tablesp water

Instructions:

- Place the chocolate and walnuts in a food processor and process them until the powder is fine.
- Add all the remaining ingredients except water and mix until the mixture forms a ball Depending on the consistency of the mixture, you may or may not have to apply the water- you don't want it to be too messy.

- Form the mixture into bite-sized balls using your hands, and refrigerate for at least 1 hour in an airtight container before eating them. In some more cocoa or desiccated coconut you could roll some of the balls to achieve a different finish, if you like. They will keep it in your fridge for up to 1 week.

Sirt Super Salad

Servings: 1

Ingredients:

- 1/2 cup avocado, peeled, stoned, and sliced
- 1 tblespoon extra virgin olive oil
- juice of 1/4 lemon
- 1/2 cup celery including leaves, sliced
- 1/8 cup red onion, sliced
- 1 3/4 oz (50g) arugula
- 1 3/4 oz (50g) endive leaves
- 3 1/2 oz (100g) smoked salmon slices
- 1/8 cups (15g) walnuts, chopped
- 1 tablespoon capers
- 1 large Medjool date, pitted and chopped
- 1/4 cup (10g) parsley, chopped

Instructions

- Place the leaves of salad on a plate, or in a large bowl.
- Mix all the remaining ingredients and serve over the leaves.

Sirtfood Diet's Shakshuka

Servings: 1
Prep Time: 0 hours 40 mins
Cook Time: 0 hours 0 mins
Total Time: 0 hours 40 mins

Ingredients

- 30 g Kale, remove stems and roughly chopped
- 1 tsp. Groud cumin
- 1 tsp. Ground turmeric
- 1 tbsp. Chopped parsley
- 2 Medium eggs
- 1 tsp. Paprika
- 1 tsp. Extra virgin olive oil
- 40 g Red onion, finely chopped
- 1 Garlic clove, finely chopped
- 30 g Celery, finely chopped
- 1 Bird's eye chilli, finely chopped
- 400 g Tinned chopped tomatoes

Instructions

- Heat over medium–low heat, a small, deep-sided frying pan. Add the oil and fry for 1–2

minutes the onion, garlic, celery, chilli, and
spices.

- Adding the tomatoes, then leave the sauce to
simmer gently, stirring occasionally for 20
minutes.

- Stir in the kale then cook for another 5
minutes. If you're feeling the sauce gets too
thick, just add a bit of water. Stir in the
parsley, if your sauce has a nice rich
consistency.

- Bring in the sauce two small wells, and crack
each egg into them. Reduce heat to its lowest
setting and use a lid or foil to cover the pan.
Leave the eggs for 10–12 minutes to cook,
where the whites should be firm while the
yolks are still runny. Cook for an additional 3–
4 minutes, if you prefer firm yolks. Serve right
away-ideally straight from the oven.

Green Bean, Tomato and Almond Stir Fry

Servings: 4

Ingredients

- Zest and juice of half a lemon
- 1 tbsp of tamari
- 2 tbsp olive oil
- 1 tsp root ginger, finely chopped
- 2 tomatoes, chopped
- 2 tbsp almonds, toasted
- Salt and pepper
- A handful of basil leaves
- 1 clove of garlic, finely chopped
- 450g/1lb of green beans eg: French beans, Runner beans, and Sugar Snap Peas, sliced into 2cm lengths.
- A dash of toasted sesame oil

Instructions

- Inside a saucepan heat the oil and add the root ginger and cook for a few minutes. Stir in the garlic then cook for one minute.
- Adding the sliced beans, lemon juice, a dash of toasted sesame oil, a tamari dash and a few tablespoons tea. Cover with a lid over the pan

and cook for 5-10 minutes until the beans are cooked. If it starts drying out, put more water after a few minutes.

- Stir in almonds, tomatoes, and lemon zest, season with salt and pepper, sprinkle on the leaves of basil and serve immediately.

Iced Coconut Matcha Latte

This matcha iced coconut latte is a powerhouse drink, it fills you with energy and keeps you happy for ages! It tastes so delicious and is the perfect replacement for shop-bought sugar-filled iced lattes and frappes!

Servings: 1 large glass

Ingredients

- 2 teaspoons matcha powder
- Big handful of ice, divided into 3
- 250ml coconut milk
- 1 tspoon maple syrup or 2 drops stevia
- 175ml nut milk (almond/cashew are best)
- 1 teaspoon coconut oil
- ¼ teaspoon vanilla powder
- Pinch of pink Himalayan or sea salt
- 1 teaspoon maca powder (optional)

Instructions

- Put/place all ingredients in a blender except coconut milk and 1/3 of ice, and blend until smooth. Add another 1/3 of the ice and pulse several times, just to slightly break it down.

- Adding the coconut milk and the remaining ice to a glass or container and add in the green matcha slowly, so that the two don't combine fully, but produce a beautiful layered look.

Notes: If you wanted to, you would make it into a frappe by smashing the ice.

Pear Salad with Avocado, Walnuts,and Grilled Chicken

An easy pear salad with avocado, walnuts, and grilled chicken. This combo Servings: for a satisfying meal-sized salad that's perfect for pear season!

Prep Time: 20 minutes
Total Time: 20 minutes
Servings:: 2

Ingredients

- 2 slices of cooked turkey bacon
- 1/4 cup goat cheese crumbles
- 2 Tablespoons dried cranberries
- 6 cups spring mix
- 2 pears (I used Red Anjou and Green Bartlett), sliced or chopped
- 6 oz grilled chicken breast
- 2 Tablespoons chopped walnuts, raw or toasted
- 1/2 avocado, sliced or chopped into chunks

Maple Balsamic Dressing

- 1/2 cup balsamic vinegar (I used white)
- 1/4 cup olive oil
- ½ teaspoon sea salt
- 1/4
- teaspoon Italian seasoning
- 1 teaspoon maple syrup
- 1 teaspoon dijon mustard
- 1 teaspoon minced garlic

Instructions

- Cook bacon turkey and grill chicken, if you haven't already.
- Prepare dressing in a small bowl or container, whisking all the ingredients together. I like to use a jar with a lid to store any remaining dressing in the fridge in the same jar easily.
- To make salad, catch two bowls and add a spring mix base, pear slices, grilled breast chicken, bacon, goat cheese, dried cranberries, walnuts and avocado. Drizzle salad, and enjoy the desired amount of balsamic dressing!

- Notes: Cooking turkey bacon: Microwave: place slices on a microwave-safe microwave lined paper towel spot. Cover with another paper towel and then cook for 2-4 minutes at high in the microwave, using 1 minute intervals. Every microwave is different so you are going to have to experiment with that timing. You want to have the bacon cooked through and crispy enough to snap into pieces when you chop it. You can of course also cook the stove-top bacon using the instructions for the package. I like microwave cooking bacon because it's fast and I hate bacon grease popping up all over my stove.
- I enjoy using my apple cider vinegar chicken recipe for grilled chicken, but by buying grilled chicken from the grocery store you can now use whatever seasoning you want, or save time.

Nutrition Info

Calories: 587
Carbohydrates: 53g
Fiber: 11g
Sugar: 34g
Fat: 26g
Protein: 41g

Moong Dahl

Servings: 4-6

Ingredients

- 1 red onion, finely chopped
- 1-2 tsp coriander seeds
- 1-2 tsp cumin seeds
- 300g/10 ounce split mung beans (moong dahl) – soaked for a few hours preferably
- 600ml/1pt of water
- 2 tablesp/30g olive oil, butter or ghee
- 2-4 tsp fresh ginger, chopped
- 1-2 teasp turmeric
- ¼ teasp of cayenne pepper – more if you want it spicy
- Salt & black pepper to taste

Instructions

- The split mung beans are drained and rinsed. Place them in a saucepan and cover with water. Bring to the boil and then skim off any moisture that comes up. Turn the heat down, cover and simmer.
- And In the meantime, heat the oil in a saucepan and sauté the onion until tender.

- In a heavy bottomed pan, dry fry the coriander and cumin seeds until they begin to pop. Grind them in a mortar and pestle.
- Attach the ground spices and the ginger, turmeric, and cayenne pepper to the onions. Cook on a couple of minutes.
- When the mung beans are almost cooked add to them the mixture of onion and spice. Season with pepper and salt, and continue cooking for another 10 minutes.

Dill roasted mackerel with tomatoes & steamed vegetables

Servings: 2

Ingredients

- Olive oil
- A handful of dill fronds
- 2 mackerel fillets
- 1 beef tomato, finely chopped
- Salt and pepper
- Vegetables for steaming; eg; kale, carrots, chard
- Juice of one lemon.

Instructions

- Pre-heat the oven upto 220C / gas mark 7. Spray an oven-proof olive oil dish and scatter the dill fronds over it. Place the fish over it and top with the sliced tomato. Top with pepper and salt.
- Cover with foil, then bake until the fish is cooked through for 10-15 minutes.
- Steam the vegetables and eat with the fish for 5-10 minutes. Squeeze the lemon juice over/on the vegetables and the fish.

Quinoa, Edamame and Pomegranate Seed Pilaf

Servings: 4

Ingredients

- ½ cup of sun dried tomatoes
- 225g/8oz quinoa
- Salt and pepper
- 1 pomegranate
- 2 tbsp coriander, chopped
- 1 cup of frozen edamame beans
- 2 tbsp of hazelnuts
- 3 tbsp olive oil
- 1 tbsp lemon juice
- 2 tsp of tamari

Instructions

- In a bowl, put the sun-dried tomatoes, cover with water and allow to soak.
- Then rinse the quinoa and put it in a 350ml/11fl oz water saucepan and a pinch of salt. Take to boil Cover with the lid and simmer until all the water has been absorbed-about 15 minutes.
- Add the edamame beans.

- Toast the hazelnuts over gas mark 6/200C in the oven for 8 minutes.
- Drain desiccated tomatoes from the sun.
- Combine the cooked quinoa into a large bowl with the sun-dried tomatoes and hazelnuts.
- Combine the olive oil, lemon juice and tamari to make dressing. Stir this gently into the vegetables and the quinoa.
- Season with salt and pepper, and sprinkle seeds and coriander on the pomegranate.

Quinoa Risotto with Tofu and Asparagus.

Servings: 4

- 1 tsp olive oil
- 2 tsp garlic, finely chopped/minced
- 1 cup red onion, finely diced
- 1/2 cp sun-dried tomatoes, cut into thin strips
- 2 cups vegetable stock
- 2 tblsp fresh lemon juice
- 1 cup quinoa, rinsed
- 1 tblsp lemon rind
- 1/2 tsp freshly ground black pepper
- 1/2 lb asparagus, cut into 11/2 inch lengths
- 1/2 lb firm tofu, cut into 1/2 inch cubes
- 1/2 cup toasted cashews

Instructions

· Over the medium, heat the olive oil . Sauté the garlic and onion for about one minute. Add the sun-dried tomatoes and sauté for a further minute. Add the vegetable stock, lemon juice, quinoa grains, lemon zest, black pepper and tofu. Cover and simmer 15 minutes. Place asparagus on top, cover and continue cooking for a further 5 mins. Sprinkle with toasted cashews.

Nutrition Info:

Per serving (330g): 435 calories, 24 g protein, 17 g fat (3 g saturated), 48 g carbohydrates, 40 mg cholesterol, 325 mg sodium

Buckwheat Bean and Tomato Risotto

Servings: 4

Ingredients

- 2 tbsp olive oil or butter
- 2 cloves of garlic, chopped
- 225g/8oz buckwheat
- 400ml of hot water or vegetable stock
- 225g/8oz frozen broad beans
- ½ cup of sun-dried tomatoes in oil
- Juice of half a lemon
- 2 tbsp basil or coriander, chopped
- 50g/2oz almonds, toasted
- Salt and pepper

Instructions

- Inside a frying pan, heat the olive oil / butter. Add the garlic, and cook for one minute.
- Add the buckwheat to the saucepan and stir well to coat in the oil.
- Add the stock or hot water. Cover for 10 minutes, then simmer.
- Stir in the beans. Cook, until the beans are tender, for a few minutes.
- Season with salt and pepper and add the sun-dried tomatoes, lemon juice, fresh herbs, and almonds.

Asian Shrimp Stir-Fry With Buckwheat Noodles

Servings: 1

Ingredients:

- 3 oz (75g) soba (buckwheat noodles)
- 2 garlic cloves, finely chopped
- 1 Thai chili, finely chopped
- 1 tspoon finely chopped fresh ginger
- 1/8 cup (20g) red onions, sliced
- 1/3 pound shelled raw jumbo shrimp, deveined
- 2 tspoons tamari (you can use soy sauce if you are not avoiding gluten)
- 2 tspoons extra virgin olive oil
- 1/2 cup celery including leaves, trimmed and sliced, with leaves set aside
- 1/2 cup green beans, chopped
- 3/4 cup kale, roughly chopped
- 1/2 cup (100ml) chicken stock

Instructions

- · Heat up a saucepan over high heat, then cook the shrimp for 2 to 3 minutes in 1 teaspoon tamari and 1 teaspoon oil.

- · Put the shrimp onto a plate. Wipe the pan out with a towel of paper, as you will be using it again.
- · Cook the noodles for 5 minutes to 8 minutes in boiling water, or as directed on the pack. Drain and set aside.
- · Meanwhile, in the remaining tamari and oil over medium - high heat, fry the garlic, ginger, red onion, green beans, chili, celery (but not the leaves), and kale for 2-3 min. Adding the stock and bring to a boil, then cook for a minute or two until cooked but crunchy.
- · Add the shrimp, noodles, and leaves of celery to the pan, bring back to a boil, then remove and serve from heat.

Sirtfood Diet's turmeric baked salmon

Prep Time: 0 hours 10 mins
Cook Time: 0 hours 10 mins
Total Time: 0 hours 20 mins
Servings: 1

Ingredients

- 40 g Red onion, finely chopped
- 60 g Tinned green lentils
- 1 Garlic clove, finely chopped
- 1 Bire's eye chilli, finely chopped
- 150 g Celery, cut into 2cm lengths
- Skinned Salmon
- 1 tsp. Extra virgin olive oil
- 1 tsp. Ground turmeric
- 1/4 Juice of a lemon
- 1 tsp. Extra virgin olive oil
- 1 tsp. Mild curry powder
- 130 g Tomato, cut into 8 wedges
- 100 ml Chicken or vegetable stock
- 1 tbsp. Chopped parsley

Instructions

- Heat the oven to a level of 200C / gas 6.
- Begin with the spicy celery. Heat over medium-low heat a frying pan, add olive oil, then onion, garlic, ginger, chili and celery. Fry gently for 2 minutes – 3 minutes or until softened but not coloured, then add the curry powder and then cook for a minute more.
- Then add the tomatoes, stock and lentils and gently simmer for 10 minutes. Based on how crunchy you like your celery you might want to increase or decrease the cooking time.
- In the meantime, bring together the turmeric, oil and lemon juice and rub over the salmon. Set on a baking tray and cook 8–10 minutes.
- Stir the parsley through the celery to finish, and serve with salmon.

Strawberry Buckwheat Tabbouleh

Servings: 1

Ingredients:

- 1/3 cup (50g) buckwheat
- 1 tablespoon ground turmeric
- 1/2 cup (80g) avocado
- 3/8 cup (65g) tomato
- 1/8 cup (20g) red onion
- 1/8 cup (25g) Medjool dates, pitted
- 1 tablespoon capers
- 3/4 cup (30g) parsley
- 2/3 cup (100g) strawberries, hulled
- 1 tablespoon extra virgin olive oil
- juice of 1/2 lemon
- 1 ounce (30g) arugula

Instructions

- Cook the buckwheat with the turmeric as directed on the package.
- Drain to cool, and set aside.
- Chop the avocado, dates, capers, tomato, red onion, and parsley thinly and mix with the cool buckwheat.
- Slice the strawberries, and mix the oil and lemon juice gently into the salad. Serve them on an arugula bed.

Vegan Carrot Ginger Soup (Instant Pot)

Vegan Ginger Carrot Soup made in the Instant Pot, or on top of your stove. A simple and healthy soup recipe in minutes to have at your table!

Prep Time 10 mins
Cook Time 15 mins
Total Time 25 mins
Servings: 4 -6

Ingredients

- 2 tablespoons ginger finely chopped
- 5 cups carrots peeled & chopped
- 900 mL vegetable broth
- 3/4 teaspoons salt
- 1/2 teaspoon pepper
- 1 teaspoon dried thyme leaves
- 1 tablespoon olive oil
- 1 onion chopped
- 2 cloves garlic minced
- 1 can 400mL/ 13.5 oz coconut milk
- juice of 1/2 lime

Instructions

Instant Pot

- Cook onion in olive oil for 5 minutes-6 minutes using the sauté feature on your Instant Pot.

- Add the garlic & ginger and cook for 1-2 minutes. Switch off the feature sauté.
- To combine, add the carrots, stock, salt and pepper and stir. Put the lid on, turn the vent to' seal' and cook for 5 minutes at manually high pressure.
- After time is up do a quick release of pressure.
- Blend in with an immersion blender until smooth.
- Add coconut and lime juice, and enjoy!

Stove Top.

- Cook the onion over medium heat in olive oil for 5-6 minutes.
- Add the garlic & ginger and cook for 1-2 minutes.
- Add the carrots, stock, salt, pepper, and thyme and combine to stir. Cook until the carrots are soft, for 20-30 minutes.
- Blend in with an immersion blender until smooth.
- Add coconut and lime juice, and enjoy!

Nutrition Info

Calories: 200kcal, Fat: 13g, Saturated Fat: 9g, Carbohydrates: 13g, Protein: 8gSodium: 462mg, Fiber: 3g, Sugar: 7g

Aromatic Chicken Breast With Kale & Red Onions And A Tomato And Chili Salsa

Servings: 1

Ingredients:

- juice of 1/4 lemon
- 1 tablespoon extra virgin olive oil
- 3/4 cup (50g) kale, chopped
- 1/8 cup (20g) red onion, sliced
- 1/4 poundskinless, boneless chicken breast
- 2 tspns ground turmeric
- 1 teaspoon chopped fresh ginger
- 1/3 cup (50g) buckwheat

For The Salsa

- 1 medium tomato (130g)
- 2 tablespoons (5g) parsley, finely chopped
- juice of 1/4 lemon
- 1 Thai chili, finely chopped
- 1 tablespoon capers, finely chopped

Instructions

- Remove the eye from the tomato to make the salsa, and chop it very fine, taking care to keep the liquid as much as possible. Mix/combine with the chili, capers, lemon juice and parsley. You might put it all in a blender but the end result is a little different.

- Heat the oven to 220 ° C (425oF). In 1 teaspoon of turmeric, the lemon juice, and a little oil, marinate the chicken breast. Turn on for five to ten minutes.
- Heat the oven-proof frying pan until hot, then add the marinated chicken and cook on each side for about a min or so until pale golden, then transfer to the oven (set on a baking tray if your pan is not oven-proof) for 8 to 10 minutes or until cooked. Remove from the oven, cover with foil, then leave for 5 minutes to rest before serving.
- Meanwhile, boil the kale for 5 minutes in a steamer. Fry the red onions & the ginger in a little oil, then add the cooked kale and fry for another minute until soft but not browned.
- Cook the buckwheat with the remaining turmeric tablespoon, as per package instructions. Serve with chicken, vegetables, and salsa.

Miso-Marinated Baked Cod With Stir-Fried Greens & Sesame

Servings: 1

Ingredients:

- 3 1/2 teaspoons (20g) miso
- 1 tablespoon mirin
- 1 tablespoon extra virgin olive oil
- 1 x 7-ounce (200g) skinless cod fillet
- 1/8 cup (20g) red onion, sliced
- 1 tbspoon tamari (or soy sauce, if not avoiding gluten)
- 1/4 cup (40g) buckwheat
- 1 Thai chili, finely chopped
- 1 teaspoon finely chopped fresh ginger
- 1 teaspoon ground turmeric
- 3/8 cup (40g) celery, sliced
- 2 garlic cloves, finely chopped
- 3/8 cup (60g) green beans
- 3/4 cup (50g) kale, roughly chopped
- 1 teaspoon sesame seeds
- 2 tablespoons (5g) parsley, roughly chopped

Instructions

- Mix the 1 teaspoon. of oil with the miso, and mirin Rub the cod all over, and leave for 30 minutes to marinate. Heat the oven to 220 ° C (425oF).
- Bake the cod for about 10 minutes.
- Meanwhile, heat the remaining oil to a large frying pan or wok. Stir-fry the onion for a few minutes, then add the celery, garlic, chili, ginger, green beans and kale. Toss and fry until the kale is cooked through and tender. To help the cooking process you might need to add a little water to the pan.
- Cook the buckwheat along with the turmeric according to the package instructions.
- To the stir-fry add the sesame seeds, parsley, and tamari and serve with buckwheat and fish.

CONCLUSION

If you are dead set to try the Sirtfood Diet, experiment first by incorporating more of the signature staples of the diet into what you already eat at home. Incorporating foods that are rich in polyphenols, including those on the sirtfood list, can help prevent or reduce inflammatory diseases such as cardiovascular disease. Skip the initial restrictive steps and prescribed green juices, instead choose to add in antioxidant-rich foods to your eating plan in a way that you enjoy.